Disaster Bioethics: Normative Issues When Nothing is Normal

Public Health Ethics Analysis

Volume 2

Edited by

Dónal P. O'Mathúna
Bert Gordijn
Mike Clarke

During the 21st Century, Public Health Ethics has become one of the fastest growing subdisciplines of bioethics. This is the first Book Series dedicated to the topic of Public Health Ethics. It aims to fill a gap in the existing literature by providing thoroughgoing, book-length treatment of the most important topics in Public Health Ethics—which have otherwise, for the most part, only been partially and/or sporadically addressed in journal articles, book chapters, or sections of volumes concerned with Public Health Ethics. Books in the series will include coverage of central topics in Public Health Ethics from a plurality of disciplinary perspectives including: philosophy (e.g., both ethics and philosophy of science), political science, history, economics, sociology, anthropology, demographics, law, human rights, epidemiology, and other public health sciences. Blending analytically rigorous and empirically informed analyses, the series will address ethical issues associated with the concepts, goals, and methods of public health; individual (e.g., ordinary citizens' and public health workers') decision making and behaviour; and public policy. Inter alia, volumes in the series will be dedicated to topics including: health promotion; disease prevention; paternalism and coercive measures; infectious disease; chronic disease; obesity; smoking and tobacco control; genetics; the environment; public communication/trust; social determinants of health; human rights; and justice. A primary priority is to produce volumes on hitherto neglected topics such as ethical issues associated with public health research and surveillance; vaccination; tuberculosis; malaria; diarrheal disease; lower respiratory infections; drug resistance; chronic disease in developing countries; emergencies/disasters (including bioterrorism); and public health implications of climate change.

For further volumes:
http://www.springer.com/series/10067

Dónal P. O'Mathúna • Bert Gordijn
Mike Clarke
Editors

Disaster Bioethics: Normative Issues When Nothing is Normal

Normative Issues When Nothing is Normal

Springer

Editors
Dónal P. O'Mathúna
Dublin City University
Dublin
Ireland

Mike Clarke
Queen's University Belfast
Belfast
Northern Ireland

Bert Gordijn
Dublin City University
Dublin
Ireland

ISSN 2211-6680 ISSN 2211-6699 (electronic)
ISBN 978-94-007-3863-8 ISBN 978-94-007-3864-5 (eBook)
DOI 10.1007/978-94-007-3864-5
Springer Dordrecht Heidelberg London New York

Library of Congress Control Number: 2013950792

Printed on acid-free paper

Springer is part of Springer Science+Business Media (www.springer.com)

Contents

Part I Healthcare Ethics and Disasters

1 **Disaster Bioethics: An Introduction** 3
Dónal P. O'Mathúna, Bert Gordijn and Mike Clarke

2 **Macro-triage in Disaster Planning** 13
Henk Ten Have

3 **Ethics and Emergency Disaster Response. Normative Approaches and Training Needs for Humanitarian Health Care Providers** 33
Lisa Schwartz, Matthew Hunt, Lynda Redwood-Campbell and Sonya de Laat

4 **Triage in Disaster Medicine: Ethical Strategies in Various Scenarios** 49
Y. Michael Barilan, Margherita Brusa and Pinchas Halperin

5 **When Relief Comes from a Different Culture: Sri Lanka's Experience of the Asian Tsunami** 65
Athula Sumathipala

6 **Ethical Issues in Health Communications: Strategies for the (Inevitable) Next Pandemic** 77
Joseph Scanlon

7 **Evidence and Healthcare Needs During Disasters** 95
Aasim Ahmad, Syed Mamun Mahmud and Dónal P. O'Mathúna

Part II Research Ethics and Disasters

8 **Interests Divided: Risks to Disaster Research Subjects vs. Benefits to Future Disaster Victims** 109
Evelyne Shuster

9 Purple Dinosaurs and Victim Consent to Research in Disasters 129
George J. Annas

10 Setting Disaster Research Priorities 143
Virginia Murray and Anthony Kessel

11 Studying Vulnerable Populations in the Context of Enhanced Vulnerability 159
Ruth Macklin

12 Research Ethics Governance in Disaster Situations 175
Doris Schopper

13 Ethical Concerns in Disaster Research—A South African Perspective 191
Keymanthri Moodley

Appendix I—Code of Conduct for the International Red Cross and Red Crescent Movement and NGOs in Disaster Relief 205

Appendix II—WMA Statement on Medical Ethics in the Event of Disasters 207

Index 211

Contributors

Aasim Ahmad Aga Khan University, Karachi, Pakistan

George J. Annas Boston University, Boston, USA

Y. Michael Barilan Department of Medical Education, Sackler School of Medicine, Tel Aviv University, Tel Aviv, Israel

Margherita Brusa Department of Pediatrics, University of Padua, Padua, Italy

Mike Clarke Queen's University Belfast, Belfast, Northern Ireland

Sonya de Laat McMaster University, Hamilton, Canada

Bert Gordijn Dublin City University, Dublin, Ireland

Pinchas Halperin Tel Aviv Medical Center, Tel Aviv, Israel

Matthew Hunt McGill University, Montreal, Canada

Anthony Kessel Public Health England, London, UK

Ruth Macklin Albert Einstein College of Medicine, Bronx, New York, USA

Syed Mamun Mahmud The Kidney Centre Post Graduate Training Institute, Karachi, Pakistan

Keymanthri Moodley Stellenbosch University, Tygerberg, South Africa

Virginia Murray Public Health England, London, UK

Dónal P. O'Mathúna Dublin City University, Dublin, Ireland

Lynda Redwood-Campbell McMaster University, Hamilton, Canada

Joseph Scanlon Carleton University, Ottawa, Canada

Doris Schopper Center for Education and Research in Humanitarian Action, University of Geneva, Geneva, Switzerland

Lisa Schwartz McMaster University, Hamilton, Canada

Evelyne Shuster Veterans Affairs Medical Center, Philadelphia, USA

Athula Sumathipala King's College, London, UK

Henk Ten Have Duquesne University, Pittsburgh, USA

Part I
Healthcare Ethics and Disasters

Chapter 1
Disaster Bioethics: An Introduction

Dónal P. O'Mathúna, Bert Gordijn and Mike Clarke

1.1 Disasters

Most disasters are characterised by sudden onset, overwhelming needs and insufficient resources. Recent examples have revealed their devastation graphically, including the 2011 Great East Japan earthquake and tsunami, the 2010 and 2011 flooding in Pakistan, the 2010 earthquake in Haiti, Hurricane Katrina in the US in 2005, and the 2004 Indian Ocean tsunami.

While large-scale disasters receive widespread attention, smaller disasters occur regularly, averaging one per day. According to the United Nations International Strategy for Disaster Reduction (UNISDR), 2010 was the deadliest year for disasters in decades: 373 natural disasters killed 300,000 people, impacted 200 million more, and cost over US$100 billion (UNISDR 2011a). Foremost amongst the deadliest of these disasters were the Haitian earthquake that killed over 222,000 people and a heat wave that killed 56,000 people in Russia. Subsequently, 2011 was the costliest year ever for damages from disasters, estimated at between US$350 and 380 billion, largely due to the Japanese earthquake (McClean 2012).

The increased impact of disasters has happened for a number of reasons. Foremost among these are climate change and increased urbanisation involving poor planning and bad building practices (IFRC 2010). Although low- and middle-income countries suffer the greatest loss of life from disasters, high-income countries experience the greatest disaster-related economic losses. Thus, while the impact of disasters varies by country, it is consistently highly significant. As a result, disaster preparedness and risk reduction are top priorities for the United Nations (UN) and many other organisations.

D. P. O'Mathúna (✉)
Dublin City University, Dublin, Ireland
e-mail: donal.omathuna@dcu.ie

B. Gordijn
Dublin City University, Dublin, Ireland

M. Clarke
Queen's University Belfast, Belfast, Northern Ireland

D. P. O'Mathúna et al. (eds.), *Disaster Bioethics: Normative Issues When Nothing is Normal,* Public Health Ethics Analysis 2, DOI 10.1007/978-94-007-3864-5_1,

Disasters are defined in various ways, as will be apparent in the chapters of this book. While the specific details vary, a number of common characteristics are recognised by various sources. Foremost among these are that local, and often national, capacity to respond is overwhelmed which creates immense logistical problems as well as leading to a host of ethical dilemmas. The World Medical Association (WMA) highlights a number of features common to disasters (WMA 2006):

- Sudden, unexpected onset requiring prompt response
- Massive damage to materials, infrastructure, and the environment
- Large numbers of human casualties, with difficulties accessing survivors
- Complications to relief efforts from weather, pollution, infection and psychological factors
- Insecurity due to physical dangers, conflict or violence
- Broad media attention.

Disasters are usually categorised into one of three groups: natural disasters (such as floods, earthquakes, or mudslides), human-related disasters (such as industrial and transportation accidents, as well as disasters due to war or terrorism), or complex emergencies, which involve natural and human causes. These classifications point to some of the major general causes of disasters. However, such classifications can be arbitrary, especially as both natural and human-related factors are involved in most disasters.

1.2 Disaster Bioethics

Disasters involve many complex issues. There is a growing realisation that amongst these, ethical issues are frequently involved. In October 2011, at the second meeting of the European Forum for Disaster Risk Reduction (EFDRR 2011), the Council of Europe committed itself to a new framework for disaster risk reduction. In this, ethics was held to be crucial to putting people first in disaster risk reduction. The first recommendation was to address the ethical aspects of disaster risk reduction through the application of ethical principles. However, specific details were not provided about the ethical framework to be used, or how the ethical issues could, or should, be addressed.

Ethics is a vast subject, broadly covering issues of right and wrong in human behaviour, attitudes, character and policy. This book will not attempt to provide a theoretical foundation for ethics or disaster bioethics. Such work is only beginning, and much philosophical reflection remains to occur in this area (Zack 2010). This book is a contribution to the field of applied ethics. Rather than propose one particular approach to resolving ethical issues in disasters, this book seeks to draw attention to the many ethical issues. Our aim is that ethicists and disaster responders will see the need to apply various ethical frameworks and approaches to the ethical issues in disasters. Different chapters show how this already has been attempted. One conclusion already arising is that much contemporary western bioethics has important limitations when applied in disaster settings (Karadag and Hakan 2012). One of the reasons for this is the way resources (and people) are completely overwhelmed in disasters. Another is that contemporary bioethics is very focused on individuals and individual rights, while disasters lead to a greater focus on the rights and care of populations. As such, disaster bioethics addresses issues raised within public health ethics, itself a fledging field of bioethics (Lee et al. 2012).

Widespread agreement exists that ethical issues occur throughout disaster management and response (Jensen 1997). High-level statements on disaster ethics exist. The International Federation of Red Cross and Red Crescent Societies (IFRC) has a Code of Conduct for disaster responders (IFRC 1994), which is reprinted by permission in Appendix I. In 2006 the World Medical Association issued a *Statement on medical ethics in the event of disasters* (WMA 2006), which is reprinted by permission in Appendix II.

However, such statements can be seen as highly aspirational and would require further exploration to permit practical application. After all, numerous ethical decisions must be made in disaster preparation, and also during responses. But these decisions are highly complex, involve much uncertainty and risk, and in disasters are made in the midst of chaotic and often dangerous situations. Often the decisions involve trying to choose the 'lesser evil', rather than finding an ideal solution (Magone et al. 2011). Such difficulties create challenges for those seeking to address ethical issues in disasters.

For example, in the immediate aftermath of disasters, healthcare professionals may have to decide who they accept into care and who they must turn away. Such triage decisions are difficult, especially knowing that in other circumstances they could probably help the injured survive. Once in care, decisions must be made about how best to treat patients, especially knowing that follow-up care may be inadequate, if not non-existent. Further triage decisions must be made when considering whether treatment should be withdrawn from existing patients to care for potential patients (Eyal and Firth 2012). Using medical criteria to make triage decisions is one thing, but other factors lead to complications. Pressure can be brought to bear to take care of certain people because they have powerful connections, or to give others lower priority for non-medical reasons.

Other ethical dilemmas arise when professionals are asked to practice in ways they know they are not credentialed for 'at home.' Disagreements arise between personnel, as they do in all areas of practice, but they seem accentuated by the environment. Local customs and practices may appear to go against evidence-based practice, creating dilemmas over what should be done or recommended. Different approaches may seem warranted on the ground, but be contrary to 'head office' guidelines. Organisations may have commitments and obligations to governments and donors that appear to conflict with meeting the needs of people in the locally affected community. When armed conflict is added on top of these, dilemmas are further intensified.

Disaster bioethics is a field of recent interest that falls within the broader area of applied ethics. While ethical dilemmas have existed throughout the history of humanitarian relief, they have rarely been examined in detail (Magone et al. 2011). Some qualitative research has identified ethical dilemmas facing healthcare responders and disaster researchers. These situations can lead to moral distress, which sometimes incapacitates responders, hinders them returning to the field, or leads to long-term psychological problems (Alexander and Klein 2009). In spite of these challenges, healthcare responders are provided little training or guidance for the ethical dilemmas they face (Schwartz et al. 2010).

Disaster bioethics examines issues of moral conduct, questions of right and wrong, as encountered by individuals and organisations as they respond to the needs of people impacted by disasters. Many of these questions arise in the context of healthcare needs and provision. In addition, because these needs lead to research on how best to intervene, disaster bioethics also studies the ethical issues arising from conducting research in disaster settings. Disaster research covers a wide variety of study types, ranging from surveys asking people about their experiences and needs, to randomised controlled trials of medical interventions. Various types of studies raise different ethical issues, with some people questioning whether certain types of research should not be conducted at all during disasters. They would argue that the focus, at least during the acute phase, should be exclusively on search and rescue, and taking care of survivors.

However, decisions are made at all stages of disaster relief about what interventions or strategies to adopt. Disaster relief agencies and those developing policies for disaster risk reduction are increasingly called upon to make evidence-based decisions. Yet the available evidence is far from ideal. The Hyogo Framework for Action (HFA) is the UNISDR's plan for disaster risk reduction that details the work necessary to reduce losses from disasters. Its 2011 mid-term review noted that 'much of the existing operational research related to emergencies and disasters lacks consistency, is of poor reliability and validity and is of limited use for establishing baselines, defining standards, making comparisons or tracking trends' (UNISDR 2011b, p. 46). Hence, more research is needed to understand disasters and the best ways to reduce their risks and improve responses.

As with any research involving human subjects and participants, intricate ethical issues arise in disaster research. However, it might be especially challenging to uphold strict ethical standards in the circumstances that surround and arise from a disaster. Previous reviews of disaster responses have identified unethical research practices (Sumathipala and Siribaddana 2005) and in a small number of cases, international controversy has arisen. In other cases, participants in disaster research have not been treated respectfully, leaving them with a negative view of research (Pittaway et al. 2010). It is imperative that ethical principles be upheld in all disaster research. Ethical lapses in this area can hamper efforts to conduct further important research that might benefit both those affected by the immediate disaster and those affected by future disasters.

Disaster research in general can be justified ethically given that it may provide results that benefit future victims of disasters. However, each individual study needs to be ethically justified and demonstrate that it will be carried out to the highest possible ethical standards. Yet no internationally agreed guidelines or ethics codes exist for research in disaster settings. A working group set up after the 2004 Indian

Ocean Tsunami has developed draft guidelines for disaster research (Sumathipala et al. 2010). Médecins Sans Frontières (MSF) has developed processes to ethically review their disaster research projects (Schopper et al. 2009). However, much further work is needed to examine the ethical complexities involved in disaster research, including how to address the urgency of disaster research, the vulnerability of disaster survivors, and issues of informed consent. Several of these issues are explored in Part II of this book.

1.3 Chapter Outline

This book is divided into two parts. The first examines some of the ethical issues in responding to healthcare needs during disasters. The second examines research ethics in disaster settings. The chapters are developed from presentations given in 2011 at a symposium at the Brocher Foundation in Geneva, Switzerland.[1] The presentations and discussions highlighted many of the complex ethical dilemmas faced during disasters, and the need for further scholarly work and policy-development in this area. This book does not attempt to address all the ethical issues in disasters, nor does it provide the final word on the topics addressed. Instead, it aims to stimulate further discussion and debate on these important ethical issues.

Part I examines the ethical issues in providing health care during disasters. Henk Ten Have examines disaster bioethics from a macro-ethical perspective. He analyses ethical questions associated with the current framework of disaster relief and humanitarian aid. He examines the language used to describe disasters, and questions the legitimacy of distinguishing natural from man-made disasters. Such language has important ethical implications as it suggests certain views of human causation and responsibility. This chapter also examines recent changes in the use of military resources in disaster relief. The moral reasoning behind humanitarian action points to certain moral responsibilities: to protect populations, save lives, and relieve suffering. Ten Have argues that instead of the language of needs and compassion, humanitarianism would be better served by the language of human rights and dignity.

Healthcare professionals who have provided humanitarian health aid after disasters were interviewed by Lisa Schwartz and colleagues. Their chapter discusses some of the insights gained about the ethical challenges faced by these professionals. The interviews show how clinical decision-making in disaster contexts is complicated by factors such as resource scarcity, security conflicts and disparate cultural expectations. Because of the ethical challenges in responding to patients, professionals perceived that they were unable to provide appropriate standards of care, which

[1] Funding was provided by the Brocher Foundation (http://www.brocher.ch), Porticus UK (http://www.porticusuk.com/), the Cochrane Collaboration's Evidence Aid Project (http://www.evidenceaid.org/), and Dublin City University (http://www.dcu.ie) to bring together scholars and international organisations to discuss the ethical challenges in disasters. The editors express their thanks to these organisations for funding the symposium which permitted the discussions leading to this volume.

had profound impact on the healthcare professionals, leading to stress and burn-out. The authors conclude that training and other resources are needed to help disaster responders develop skills for managing moral dilemmas before they enter the field. The chapter proposes strategies, both theoretical and practical that may help prepare humanitarian healthcare providers to manage ethical conflicts that threaten to interfere with care.

One of the ethical dilemmas faced by healthcare professionals is the requirement to decide which of the injured to treat and not treat, or treat differently. Such triage decisions are a source of significant moral distress for healthcare professions. Michael Barilan and colleagues give an outline for triage in mass-casualty disasters. They make a distinction between three types of disasters: those impacting well-ordered societies, those that wreak havoc on the infrastructure of the society, and 'double disasters' that ravage societies whose infrastructure had already been substantially deficient because of poverty. Three schemes of triage are also examined. Each is shown to be ethically justifiable, though with each being more applicable to particular disaster scenarios. They explain their preference for the third approach that combines elements of the first two.

Many disasters involve international assistance and bring together different cultures that might otherwise have limited or difficult interactions. In his chapter, Athula Sumathipala addresses some of the ethical issues that arise in disasters because of cultural differences. Drawing on his direct experience of the response to the 2004 Tsunami in Sri Lanka, Sumathipala explores such ethical dilemmas, particularly when pre-existing cultural conflicts exist in a disaster-impacted region. The chapter proposes a number of ethical responsibilities for disaster responders in their approach to cultural differences and conflicts during disasters.

Joseph Scanlon examines ethical issues in communications during health emergencies and pandemics. Drawing from historical examples of disasters, he identifies several principles for effective and ethical communication during disasters. Planning and training are essential for effective communications to ensure responses are not made ad hoc. During a major health disaster, communications should be handled by all who have relevant and credible backgrounds, not just the healthcare community. Most elements of crisis communications can and should be anticipated in prior planning. The messages themselves should be consistent and be repeated. The information should be accurate, positive and show concern and empathy. All channels of communication should be used. Scanlon points out that communications about ethical controversies arising during disasters has received little attention. He concludes with some suggestions about how these could be addressed appropriately.

The final chapter in the first part of the book examines issues of evidence and healthcare needs during disasters. Aasim Ahmad and colleagues examine how evidence-based practice has developed within medicine, and is increasingly called for to guide humanitarian responses. They note that basing humanitarian responses on evidence-based principles is challenging and has met with resistance. However, they defend the view that generating and using evidence in disasters is ethically justified. They cite a number of myths about disasters and disaster responses, which have been overturned as better evidence is made available from disaster research. At the same time, the studies needed to develop an evidence base raise challenges for research ethics, which is the focus of Part II of the book.

The second part begins with an examination of the harms and benefits of disaster research. Evelyne Shuster argues that conducting research on people after disasters is a luxury. People should not be used merely as means to achieve other people's goals. Shuster acknowledges that many types of research can be conducted after disasters, and her focus is on clinical research that puts subjects at risk of physical harm. She claims that such research is difficult to justify in the immediate aftermath of a disaster, although it may be ethically acceptable during the recovery phase. Researchers may believe that new treatments must be tested to improve current practices and reduce the risk of harm in future disasters. However, Shuster argues that in disaster contexts combining medical care with medical research complicates the validity of informed consent and compromises the risk-benefit calculation. The risks of eroding particular moral values in the pursuit of scientific progress make such progress not worth having.

George Annas examines a recent trend that emphasises the benefit of medical research for future patients and society in general. According to Annas, this takes the emphasis off the rights of research subjects, especially regarding informed consent and the right to withdraw. Recent revelations about US medical research in Guatemala in the 1940s provide another example of medical necessity being used to over-rule human rights, with unethical results. Annas notes that the pressures and urgency of conducting disaster research could likewise lead to calls to conduct such research without consent. Ethical violations have occurred in US-sponsored research conducted in response to health disasters in Africa. If subjects' consent cannot be obtained for disaster research, Annas holds that such research should not be done. Disasters are opportunities to help victims, and should not be used as opportunities to exploit victims by doing research on them without their consent. He argues that ample opportunities exist to conduct ethically sound research without resorting to research without consent.

The next chapter explores the ethical issues involved in setting disaster research priorities. Virginia Murray and Anthony Kessel describe the difficulties and complexities involved in setting priorities for disaster research. However, overcoming these challenges is vital both to produce credible evidence for disaster risk reduction and planning, and to facilitate improved responses to humanitarian and health catastrophes. They note that little has been written on how to set disaster research priorities, and even less on the relevant ethical issues. Identifying the priorities depends partly on the systems that exist within countries, regions and international organisations. They describe three broad approaches to setting disaster research priorities and explore each critically, examining their advantages and disadvantages. They conclude by identifying the ethical issues involved in each approach and make recommendations for future planning.

Survivors of disasters are sometimes viewed as a vulnerable population when considered as research subjects. Ruth Macklin notes that being vulnerable does not, in and of itself, raise the level of risk in a research study. However, vulnerable subjects deserve additional protections, even in less risky research. Ethical guidelines often note the need for additional safeguards for vulnerable subjects, but rarely specify what such protections should be. Different types of disasters may call for different safeguards depending on the type of disaster, proximity in time to the disaster, the severity of injury or trauma, and other factors. The types of safeguards needed for vulnerable subjects in research conducted during or after a disaster will depend on contextual factors that cannot be specified in advance. Macklin describes a 'layers' approach to vulnerability that provides guidance on protections for the rights and welfare of subjects. A cardinal ethical principle is that research should never interfere with or delay medical care or other aid being provided to treat or prevent further harm to disaster victims.

Doris Schopper notes increased awareness of the need to have clear guidance for ethical review of disaster research, and that internationally accepted guidelines are lacking. General research ethics guidelines provide some direction, but are not specifically targeted at disaster research. She examines in depth the Ethics Review Board (ERB) of Médecins Sans Frontières (MSF), of which she is a member. Its governance is based on that of other research ethics guidelines. A specific procedure for pre-approval of a generic research protocol has been developed, allowing expedited approval of the finalised protocol once a disaster occurs. Schopper examines other ethical issues that can arise in disaster research, including the importance of involving the local community in disaster research, the dual use of tissue samples collected during disasters, and addressing misconceptions that research subjects may have about what it is that they are agreeing to participate in. Schopper concludes that an internationally recognised body urgently needs to develop international guidance for ethical oversight of disaster research.

South Africa has experienced few natural disasters, but has seen some man-made disasters. Keymanthri Moodley analyses South Africa's experience with HIV/AIDS and drug resistant tuberculosis as a public health disaster. While not having a sudden onset, it has created many opportunities for disaster research. When disasters occur in resource depleted settings, escalated vulnerability ensues. Moodley describes how a research ethics regulatory infrastructure and guidelines evolved rapidly in South Africa. She examines the ethical dilemmas that arose in the context of HIV/AIDS research and how these issues were addressed in ethical guidelines. She also describes how approaches to research ethics review in disaster settings are to be incorporated into South African research ethics guidelines currently under revision.

The book concludes with reprints of the 1994 IFRC *Code of Conduct* for disaster responders and the 2006 World Medical Association *Statement on medical ethics in the event of disasters*. We are grateful for permission from these organisations to reprint these statements.

As editors, we appreciate the thought and reflection that each of the contributors have put into their chapters. We offer this volume as a stimulus for further discussion. We invite interested readers to engage with these issues and contribute to the development of this new field. Our hearts and prayers go out to those hit by disasters and to the many men and women who go to their aid. Our hope is that by providing clearer ethical reflection and guidance their lives will, in some small way, be improved. Disaster bioethics is ultimately about promoting good ethical norms when nothing else seems normal. Disasters may destroy many things, but they should not destroy human dignity. *Disaster Bioethics* aims to identify ethical means to promote human dignity in the midst of disasters.

June 2013
Dublin, Ireland

References

Alexander, David A., and Susan Klein. 2009. First responders after disasters: A review of stress reactions, at-risk, vulnerability, and resilience factors. *Prehospital and Disaster Medicine* 24: 87–94.

European Forum for Disaster Risk Reduction. 2011. Second meeting of the European forum for disaster risk reduction (EFDRR). http://www.preventionweb.net/english/professional/trainings-events/events/v.php?id=22169. Accessed 20 March 2012.

Eyal, Nir, and Paul Firth. 2012. Repeat triage in disaster relief: Questions from Haiti. *PLoS Currents Disasters*. doi:10.1371/4fbbdec6279ec.

International Federation of Red Cross and Red Crescent Societies. 1994. Code of conduct. http://www.ifrc.org/en/publications-and-reports/code-of-conduct/. Accessed 20 March 2012.

International Federation of Red Cross and Red Crescent Societies. 2010. World disasters report 2010—Urban risk. http://www.ifrc.org/en/publications-and-reports/world-disasters-report/wdr2010/. Accessed 20 June 2013.

Jensen, Eva, ed. 1997. Disaster management ethics. Department of Humanitarian Affairs of the General Secretariat of the United Nations for the Disaster Management Training Program. http://reliefweb.int/report/world/disaster-management-ethics. Accessed 20 June 2013.

Karadag, C. Ozge, and A. Kerim Hakan. 2012. Ethical dilemmas in disaster medicine. *Iranian Red Crescent Medical Journal* 14 (10):602–612.

Lee, Lisa M., Charles H. Heilig, and Angela White. 2012. Ethical justification for conducting public health surveillance without patient consent. *American Journal of Public Health* 102 (1):38–44.

Magone, Claire, Michaël Neuman, and Fabrice Weissman, eds. 2011. *Humanitarian negotiations revealed: The MSF experience*. London: Hurst & Company.

McClean, Denis. 2012. Heavy disaster losses for insurance companies in 2011. http://www.unisdr.org/archive/24588. Accessed 20 March 2012.

Pittaway, Eileen, Linda Bartolomei, and Richard Hugman. 2010. 'Stop stealing our stories': The ethics of research with vulnerable groups. *Journal of Human Rights Practice* 2:229–251.

Schopper, Doris, Ross Upshur, Francine Matthys, Jerome Amir Singh, Sunita Sheel Bandewar, Aasim Ahmad, and Els van Dongen. 2009. Research ethics review in humanitarian contexts: The experience of the independent Ethics Review Board of Médecins Sans Frontières. *PLoS Medicine* 6:e1000115.

Schwartz, Lisa, Christina Sinding, Matthew Hunt, Laurie Elit, Lynda Redwood-Campbell, Naomi Adelson, Lori Luther, Jennifer Ranford, and Sonya de Laat. 2010. Ethics in humanitarian aid work: Learning from the narratives of humanitarian health workers. *AJOB Primary Research* 1:45–54.

Sumathipala, Athula, and Sisira Siribaddana. 2005. Research and clinical ethics after the tsunami: Sri Lanka. *Lancet* 366:1418–1420.

Sumathipala, Athula, Amir Jafarey, Leonardo D. de Castro, Aasim Ahmad, Darryl Marcer, Sandya Srinivasan, Nandini Kumar, Sisira Siribaddana, Sleman Sutaryo, Anant Bhan, Dananjaya Waidyaratne, Sriyakanthi Beneragama, Chandrani Jayasekera, Sarath Edirisingha, and Chesmal Siriwardhana. Ethical issues in post-disaster clinical interventions and research: A developing world perspective. Key findings from a drafting and consensus generation meeting of the Working Group on Disaster Research and Ethics (WGDRE) 2007. 2010. *Asian Bioethics Review* 2:124–142.

United Nations International Strategy for Disaster Reduction. 2011a. Killer year caps deadly decade—reducing disaster impact is "critical" says top UN disaster official. http://www.unisdr.org/archive/17613. Accessed 20 March 2012.

United Nations International Strategy for Disaster Reduction. 2011b. Hyogo Framework for Action 2005–2015 Mid-Term Review. http://www.unisdr.org/we/inform/publications/18197. Accessed 20 March 2012.

World Medical Association. 2006. Statement on medical ethics in the event of disasters. http://www.wma.net/en/30publications/10policies/d7/index.html. Accessed 20 March 2012.

Zack, Naomi. 2010. *Ethics for disaster*. Lanham: Rowman and Littlefield.

Chapter 2
Macro-triage in Disaster Planning

Henk Ten Have

2.1 Introduction

The title of this chapter combines two notions that are unusual, at least at first sight: 'macro-triage' and 'disaster planning'. With these notions our attention will be focused on the global context in which disasters happen. Rather than prioritising needs in the midst of a disaster, we also have to prioritise which disasters require what type of response. The idea is that rather than selecting disaster victims for help we also need to select disasters for major relief, and we have to determine what the short-term and long-term goals of international assistance are. This global perspective also implies that the focus of analysis will be on the normative context rather than on the ethical problems arising in the practices of disaster relief.

In order to have a better idea of the ethical considerations that might be relevant I will begin by exploring the panorama that is presented by the notions 'macro', 'triage' and 'disaster planning'. Clarifying these notions will prepare the stage for critical examination of the normative presuppositions that are already at work before events are identified as disasters. Similarly, the moral geography of humanitarian intervention is explored. The emergence of humanitarianism as the driving force for contemporary disaster relief has produced a normative context in which action and intervention is required to save lives, to protect populations and to relief suffering. However, the moral logic of this context should be critically analysed since it is prioritising compassion over human rights and justice.

H. Ten Have (✉)
Duquesne University, Pittsburgh, USA
e-mail: tenhaveh@duq.edu

D. P. O'Mathúna et al. (eds.), *Disaster Bioethics: Normative Issues When Nothing is Normal,* Public Health Ethics Analysis 2, DOI 10.1007/978-94-007-3864-5_2,

2.2 The Panorama

2.2.1 Macro-perspective

The reference to 'macro' directs our focus onto the social background and conditions of events and cases. 'Macro-ethics' is a common, although recent notion in the field of engineering ethics (Herkert 2001; Son 2008). More than healthcare ethics, engineering ethics is used to deal with a litany of disasters such as airplane crashes, gas-tank fires, and nuclear accidents. In the face of technological failures it is important to distinguish between individual responsibility and social or organisational responsibility.

However, in healthcare ethics a similar distinction is made, following Pellegrino's suggestion that there are two modes of engagement between philosophy and medicine: philosophy *in* medicine, and philosophy *of* medicine (Pellegrino 1976). The first mode refers to the application of the traditional tools of philosophy (critical reflection, dialectical reasoning, and asking first-order questions) to some medically defined problems. In this vein we can refer to ethics *in* healthcare as the application of the tools of ethics to the problems of health care. Similarly we can focus on the ethics *in* disaster management and *in* humanitarian aid. Bioethicists can serve a useful role within these practices, help to examine the ethical dilemmas in everyday activities and contribute to resolving the problems that are defined and identified as needing attention by the professionals in the field. Ironically, this mode of engagement has itself been labelled as the engineering model of bioethics since this approach to bioethics can primarily be regarded as a sophisticated technology to make a particular set of problems manageable and controllable (Ten Have 2004).

Philosophy *of* medicine, on the other hand, examines the conceptual foundations, the ideologies and the ethos which pervade the medical realm. Medicine continuously generates philosophical issues in regard to its meaning, its nature, concepts, purposes and value to society. From a critical perspective the practical context of medicine is no longer taken for granted, but it is considered to be an object of further philosophical inquiry, transcending the narrower medical context itself and producing questions that are of wider significance to understanding ourselves. Analogously, the ethics *of* healthcare can be regarded as the critical analysis of the meaning of health care, its nature, concepts, purposes and values. Such analysis assumes that healthcare as a practical human activity has a trans-medical meaning with important implications for our self-understanding. This is exactly the 'macro'-perspective that will be developed in this chapter. Rather than analysing the ethical questions that are arising within the contemporary framework of disaster relief and humanitarian aid efforts, the focus will be on the ethical questions that are associated with the framework itself. Even if our engagement with humanitarian aid seems a priori morally unquestionable, it cannot be taken for granted.

2.2.2 Triage

The second notion to highlight is 'triage'. This is a common concept in emergency medicine. In ordinary circumstances triage will classify the wounded so that they will receive optimum care. It implies decisions regarding the order of treatment based on the urgency of need. However, triage has nowadays become an essential component in disaster relief. Disasters are characterised as situations in which the number of casualties outweighs the abilities to provide healthcare (this is in fact the main characteristic of the American College of Emergency Physicians' definition of medical disasters; see ACEP 2011). In these extraordinary circumstances triage implies that not all victims can be treated. In other words, triage or the need to prioritise is already included in the definition of a disaster.

However, there is no agreement on the ethical criteria to make such decisions (Petrini 2010; Chapter 4 of this volume). In ordinary triage the focus is on the interests of individual patients. In extraordinary circumstances, the focus is unclear; is it on survival of the greatest number of persons or on survival of persons who are most likely to survive? Even if principles are proposed to guide decisions to allocate scarce resources, it is difficult to see how they solve the ethical dilemmas; the proposed principles often present a checklist of moral points of view to take into account rather than decisional tools (Barnett et al. 2009). Some even doubt whether triage itself is ethically justified. There is no evidence that triage in a disaster setting will achieve its goals of saving more lives; the current disaster triage schema may actually worsen outcomes (Sztajnkrycer et al. 2006).

It is clear that both ordinary and extraordinary triage is operating at the level of micro-ethics, i.e. decision-making for individual persons. What do we mean, then, by 'macro-triage'? In order to unravel its meaning we must identify the perspectives that are introduced with the notion of triage.

First, triage introduces the military discourse. The concept was developed in the battlefield by Baron Larrey, surgeon-in-chief of Napoleon's armies. Larrey has been praised for his egalitarian approach; selection for treatment was based on individual need rather than military rank, nationality or social status. This did not imply that available resources were focused on the interests of the individual person in need. In fact the requirements of the war effort prevailed. This remains clear in current military directives. For example, the NATO *Handbook of Emergency War Surgery* identifies three groups of patients in thermonuclear warfare: those with minimal wounds and those with too extensive wounds will not be evacuated (they either continue as fighting soldiers or they die); only those with relatively simple injuries that require immediate surgery will be evacuated and treated. Here the focus of triage is 'salvage value': salvaging the greatest number of lives and limbs. The ultimate goal of triage is to return the greatest possible number of soldiers to combat (NATO 2011, p. 182). The same military rationale underlies the concept of minimum qualifications for survival (Lin and Anderson-Shaw 2009). Saving individual lives is not important as such but only within a broader context.

Second, triage introduces a paternalistic discourse that restrains individual freedom and human rights for the sake of the public good or the well-being of the population as a whole. In the discourse of triage, basic values are not determined in a democratic process or public deliberation but they are decided by 'authorities' who take control of the events. Such control can be legally regulated. Emergencies as well as disasters are declared by legal action, and addressed with unconventional legal responses. But even then, decisions need to be made about what to legislate first, so that the term 'legal triage' has been introduced for the construction of a legal environment in which legitimate public responses are facilitated (Hodge 2006).

The fact that the introduction of the notion 'triage' is associated with military and paternalistic discourses makes clear that a micro-perspective of allocating scarce resources and selecting victims for treatment is always guided by a macro-perspective. It is precisely this encompassing perspective and its ethical implications that we have to identify.

2.2.3 Disaster Planning

Disaster planning is an oxymoron that refers to new strategies that first have developed in the area of public health. What is meant here is disaster response planning. But instead of emphasising prevention, the focus is now on preparedness. The basic idea is that catastrophic events such as pandemics but also natural disasters cannot be prevented. However we know that one day or another we have to face them, so we need to be prepared. Over the last decade countries have invested billions in preparedness strategies, plans, departments and agencies, and special legislation (preparedness acts) has been adopted. Planning and preparedness are typically done by states (e.g. the Federal Emergency Management Agency in the US).

The emphasis on preparedness is related to the present-day tendencies to consider catastrophic threats primarily as national security threats and no longer as public health problems whether or not it concerns pandemics, bioterrorism, earthquakes or nuclear proliferation. While the rationality of prevention is linked to public health, within a security perspective on-going vigilance is required. This societal approach to threats is driven by, what Andrew Lakoff (2008) has called 'vital systems security'. Preparedness, in the politics of security, should not first of all protect the national territory or the population but the critical systems that are essential for social and economic life. This approach to security developed from the practice of civil defence in the 1950s and 1960s. Lakoff shows how the way societies were dealing with the threat of a nuclear catastrophe was gradually extended to approaching natural disasters, technological accidents, terrorist attacks and later disease epidemics. Different stages of global threats can be distinguished. In the 1980s emerging disease threats, particularly emerging viral outbreaks, were the object of concerns. In the 1990s anxiety about bioterrorism (linked to disease agents such as a possible smallpox attack) were dominant. In the 2000s the focus is more on natural disasters and pandemics. It seems that there is an ever widening range of possible threats so that preparedness now has to include 'all-hazards planning'. The policy implications of such evolving threats are clear. How can we respond at all to such wide ranging catastrophic events?

The only imaginable response is a global one. By implication, the only state agencies or departments that have the planning capacity, logistics and resources to conduct relief operations are the Departments of Defence. Non-military agencies like the United Nations or the World Health Organization (WHO) cannot accomplish this task because they don't have the logistical machinery unless provided by Member States which will take time to coordinate.

The notion of preparedness therefore brings in a specific perspective and a particular logic of action (Lakoff 2007). Only certain types of problems become visible as targets of intervention. If preparedness efforts are primarily concerned with the vital infrastructure and not with population security then the global living conditions of populations (determined by poverty and lack of basic public health infrastructure) remain outside the scope of preparedness. The only imaginable response is a global one under military supervision.

The question has been raised regarding what bioethics can contribute to this new area of disaster response planning (Berg and King 2006). Bioethicists have a lot of experience for example with complex decision-making in situations of urgency. They have also actively promoted advance care planning in end-of-life decision-making. These experiences can therefore be used in the new disaster preparedness. But these contributions all focus on micro-ethics. Indeed, an increasing range of ethical problems have been identified at the level of personal interactions between care providers and care recipients. From a macro-ethical perspective on the other hand, critical questions need to be asked about the underlying assumptions in disaster response planning and about the moral implications of notions such as disaster and preparedness.

2.3 Moral Representations

2.3.1 The Moral Geography of Disasters

Definitions and classifications of disasters differ. Definitions generally combine several elements but a basic distinction is made between natural and man-made disasters.

The International Federation of the Red Cross and Red Crescent Societies (IFRC) is developing a standardised international classification of disasters. Its *World Disaster Report* 2010 distinguishes two generic categories for disasters: natural disasters and technological disasters. The natural disasters category is divided into five sub-groups, which in turn cover 12 disaster types and more than 32 sub-types, for example biological disasters (epidemics) and geophysical disasters (earthquakes and tsunamis). The technological disasters category includes, for example, industrial accidents and transport accidents. These two categories of disasters are frequent. Over the last 10 years more than 7,000 disasters have been reported. More than 1.1 million people have died and more than 2.5 million people have been affected. The total estimated damage is enormous: 986 billion US dollars (IFRC 2010). This classification does not include war, conflict-related famines, diseases and epidemics.

Another approach is to speak about 'humanitarian disasters' or 'emergencies' and divide them into complex emergencies and natural disasters (Middleton 2010). The first category of disasters is caused by human violence (as in Somalia, Sudan, Palestine, and Congo). These are primarily political events requiring long-term assistance while popular funding will generally be limited. The relief effort will never be sufficient since progress is always endangered by renewed violence. The second category is caused by natural events such as the 2004 tsunami in the Indian Ocean, the 2010 earthquake in Haiti and the 2011 earthquake and tsunami in Japan. These natural disasters evoke widespread public sympathy and generate substantial public funding. The focus of relief efforts is usually on short-term front-line activities: food, water, shelter, and medical attention.

Both classifications identify a separate category of 'natural disasters'. These disasters have the following defining characteristics:

they are unexpected, they come as a surprise, a shock;
they cause great damage, loss, suffering and destruction, creating estrangement because people's 'homes' have been destroyed;
there is no issue of human responsibility; nobody can be blamed for the fact that the disaster has taken place since there is no human causation.

This last characteristic demarcates natural disasters from man-made ones (Clark 2005; Korf 2006). Humanitarian disasters caused by civil war for example are the result of human evil. There is a different moral responsibility. Identifying a disaster as 'natural' therefore introduces a specific moral discourse. Natural disasters create innocent, 'pure' victims. They generate a particular responsiveness; we are moved because fellow human beings are hurt and in need. Disasters nowadays have a global impact and call for our sympathy, solidarity and generosity. We are touched by personal stories of how human beings are assisting each other. The usual pattern of human interaction based on exchange and self-interest is suddenly transformed. Our world is disturbed by images of distant suffering making us aware that we are all in the same human predicament of fragility, exposing the vulnerability of human beings and inciting reciprocity and unconditional help. Natural disasters are therefore a paradigm case for humanitarian aid. They furthermore highlight the essence of ethics. What is the value of ethics if we don't care about the victims of such unfortunate events?

However, the usual distinction between natural and man-made disasters, and thus the moral geography it is introducing, is questionable. The origins of disasters can be different and some are indeed not influenced by human beings. But what makes an event into a disaster is its impact on human beings. If there would be an earthquake in a completely uninhabited area without any negative effect on humans, it will be a geophysical event but not a disaster. And in the present-day interconnected world it is difficult to see that a large-scale 'natural' disaster does not impact on human beings. But if the human impact is what makes an event disastrous, it is at the same time clear that this negative impact is often the result of prior human interventions that have created conditions of vulnerability.

A comparison of three recent earthquakes quickly shows that poorer and less developed countries are disproportionally impacted. In January 2010 Haiti was struck by an earthquake with a magnitude of 7.0. Ultimately 316,000 people were killed and 1.5 million people made homeless. The economic damage to the island was estimated at $14 billion (120 per cent of Haiti's gross domestic product). The following month, February 2010, a more severe earthquake occurred off the coast of Chile (with a magnitude of 8.8). Approximately 500 persons were killed and 370,000 homes damaged. The economic damage was estimated between $15–30 billion (10–15 per cent of Chile's GDP). Very recently, in March 2011, Japan was hit by one of the largest earthquakes ever recorded (with a magnitude of 9.0). The exact number of victims is still unknown but will be approximately 25,000 with 100,000 buildings damaged or destroyed. Regardless of the magnitude of the earthquake the disaster in Haiti was vastly more destructive and deadly. This is generally attributed to the state of development of the country. Haiti is the poorest country in the western hemisphere; 80 % of the population is living under the poverty line. The enormous number of casualties is not only due to the earthquake but to the extremely poor living conditions and the inability of the state or the population to take protective measures or even to organise relief. The example of Haiti is also ironic (Middleton 2010). The same countries that have been the first to provide humanitarian assistance were also the ones that have created the long-term conditions for the severe impact of the earthquake. Haiti used to be the richest French colony in the New World. When it declared independence as the first black republic in 1804 it had to provide exorbitant indemnities to France for the next 143 years. All the country's revenues were used to pay the former colonisers. In 1900 around 80 per cent of the national budget was used in payments to the French. In 1947 when the debt was paid off the Haitian economy was ruined, the land deforested, the population living in poverty and no infrastructure developed (Macintyre 2010). From this perspective, it is not the geophysical phenomenon that caused the disaster in Haiti but the colonial history.

Another example that demonstrates that disasters are always complex, and involve an interplay between natural processes and human activity, is Hurricane Katrina, one of the worst disasters in US history. This 2005 disaster is analysed by Byron Newberry (2010) using a macro-ethical approach. His analysis is contested since it is not evident that there is an ethical problem at all. For many, the hurricane was a natural hazard. If there have been failures in the hurricane protection system, nobody can be blamed for the devastation of New Orleans. That means that there is no problem to be discussed in terms of ethics; it is simply a technical issue. The power of nature has been so overwhelming that there is no question of negligence or irresponsible behaviour of individual engineers. The vocabulary of ethics, pointing to unethical conduct, responsibility, duties, does not apply. That may be true, Newberry agrees, but for the micro-level of interpersonal interactions. He advocates a macro-ethical point of view focusing on the complex socio-technical systems in which responsibilities are located at various levels of public policy, risk assessment and organisational behaviour. Catastrophic events do not occur as the result of unethical decisions of individuals but as the consequence of the confluence of many, seemingly insignificant decisions at various levels. Newberry shows for example how levees and floodwalls were inadequately constructed, based on wrong assumptions about possible risks. Available information that the hurricane protection system was vulnerable was simply left unused (because it endangered the uniformity of the system or was considered to be too costly). The protection system was furthermore built over a long span of time using the original specifications. However, the environment continued to change, so that the system was inadequate when it was completed. Furthermore, this was known to be the case. In spite of this, a false sense of security was created by suggesting that nature was now under human control.

The disastrous impact of the natural hazard (the hurricane) due to the vulnerabilities of human-constructed systems has, like in Haiti, a social and historical background that make quick and easy remedies unlikely. The city of New Orleans' susceptibility for disaster is the consequence of centuries of development, human engineering and political decision-making. The establishment of the city took place 300 years ago in precarious conditions, starting a long history of defending it from storms and floods. The city cannot be erased and relocated elsewhere. That means that the problem of flood protection can never be solved; it will require a never-ending, even ever-escalating effort. Problems solved somewhere will return more severely elsewhere. Channelling the river for example has allowed the economic development of land behind the levees but has made the system much more vulnerable. What is at stake is the human effort to preserve New Orleans as a major river/seaport. It is known that the Mississippi river delta is changing every 1,000 years. Human intervention is preventing the delta-switching that normally should have happened already.

This contest between human intervention and nature is in fact creating the vulnerability to disasters. The case of New Orleans resembles the case of my native country, the Netherlands. Obviously policy-makers did not want New Orleans to have the same fate as Bruges, the capital of West Flanders. The name Bruges means 'landing stage' or 'port', indicating that the city initially was a seaport. Around 1050 this access was lost due to gradual silting. But a major storm in 1134 shifting the coast line created a natural channel so that that access was restored in a different way but Bruges was now 10 miles inland. In the Netherlands, there is already a long list of 'drowned lands', settlements lost to the floods (see Wikipedia 2011). But the Dutch don't want the western, most populated half of the country to disappear into the sea. It is an uphill battle. Risks can never be excluded, even with the most perfect engineering technology. So we know, one day, another disaster will occur. But we cannot only blame nature if we continuously try to domesticate it. The interplay of natural processes and human activity implies that there always is the ethical issue of human responsibility.

2.3.2 The Moral Geography of Humanitarian Relief

A particular publicity campaign for the US navy on American TV has impressed me. You see warships and soldiers amidst devastation due to disasters such as the 2004 tsunami and the 2010 earthquake in Haiti. Once the heroic music reaches a crescendo you can read: 'America's Navy. A global force for good'. The military is nowadays one of the major providers of humanitarian assistance. Four weeks after the 2004 tsunami the White House claimed that 16,000 US troops were engaged in relief work, especially in Indonesia. After the Haiti earthquake, the US Southern Command was coordinating relief efforts. The very next day special operations military arrived in the country. One week later the hospital ship USNS Comfort dropped anchor (Etienne et al. 2010). Soon more than 22,000 military personnel were involved in the relief effort, engaging 23 US navy ships, 57 helicopters and 264 aircraft.

The present-day connection of humanitarian aid and military intervention is surprising since the so-called first phase of modern humanitarianism was initiated by the horrors of war. Henri Dunant founded in 1863 the International Committee of the Red Cross because he had witnessed the suffering of thousands of wounded soldiers who were simply abandoned at the battle of Solferino. The innovation of Dunant was not so much the creation of a system of care for victims but rather that such system was based on the moral principles of impartiality (relief is solely based on need and provided without any distinction as to nationality, race, religious beliefs, social class or political opinions) and neutrality of the care providers, so that they will be protected and respected by all parties. Dunant's ideas were soon expanded in two directions. One was that the purpose of providing humane treatment to those injured in war was generalised to providing care for all those who were suffering from floods, famines, earthquakes and epidemics and also to refugees. All those in need due to conflict or disaster will receive basic assistance with food, water, shelter and medical care. The initial ideas were expanded into a set of seven fundamental principles of the Red Cross: humanity, impartiality, neutrality, independence, voluntary service, unity and universality (Barnett and Weiss 2008). Such principles articulate the moral geography of humanitarian aid: it is by definition disinterested and purely philanthropic.

The concept of neutrality has become more and more difficult to uphold. In practice it is often violated as well as exploited for political purposes. But there are also more fundamental reasons why the primordial ethics of humanitarian assistance have been criticised (Middleton 2010).

The first reason is that international aid is explicitly regarded as an instrument of foreign policy. In 1918 US President Woodrow Wilson announced his Fourteen Points leading to a new world order with humanitarian assistance as a necessary part of foreign policy. Wilson's military occupation of Haiti, Santo Domingo, Cuba and Nicaragua were all presented as humanitarian assistance. In 1949, during the emergence of many new states, President Harry Truman launched the phenomenon of foreign aid or development assistance. The justification was moral (Hattori 2003). More developed states have an obligation to help less developed states. This will contribute to world peace and prosperity. But it also embodies the ideal of humanitarianism. If countries have basic needs and more developed countries are able to satisfy these needs, they should provide relief.

But such assistance is not disinterested. Humanitarian assistance is mostly managed by the ministries of defence and foreign affairs. Ultimately it is not idealism but self-interest of the state that prevails. In 1919 Haiti had been occupied by the US because it was heavily in debt. A system of mass forced labour was set up to make sure that the debt could be paid. The 2004 tsunami relief in Indonesia was followed by enormous arms sales a few weeks later. Foreign aid therefore has been criticised as institutionalising virtuous practices in the interests of the powerful (Hattori 2003). Its purpose is to legitimise an existing material order through transforming a material hierarchy (global injustice and social inequality) into a moral hierarchy between donor and recipient. The developed and often former colonial states have the virtue of giving, philanthropy and beneficence. Rather than emphasising the rights of recipients, humanitarian aid in this perspective only legitimises the power differences and inequalities that exist.

Secondly, the moral geography of humanitarian aid changed significantly in the 1990s after the end of the Cold War (Smith 2009). Before that time military interventions were not justified with humanitarian arguments but by the 1990s this had become a legitimate justification. Since then the number of humanitarian operations grew greatly, particularly in response to man-made catastrophes. This is due to a significant increase in the number of interstate conflicts but also to the growing influence of the idea of human rights. In fact humanitarian aid is changing into humanitarian intervention (Chatterdjee and Scheid 2003). For a long time, the military has assisted in the delivery of humanitarian aid. But since the 1990s military interventions themselves are increasingly justified as ‘humanitarian’. The major motivation for intervention is a moral one. The intervention is ‘humanitarian’ since it is not carried out for the usual military reasons but out of concern to help. Governments themselves fail to protect their citizens or are violating the human rights of their citizens. Military assistance by others is therefore necessary to protect this population even if it means that national sovereignty must be overruled. The crucial notion used in justifications is ‘rescue’: the intervention is necessary in order to rescue and protect the people in a foreign territory from gross violations of their basic human rights (Walzer 1995). The purpose is saving people from harm done by the same authorities who should protect them. British Prime Minister Blair justified (in 1999) the bombing campaign in Serbia and Kosovo: we are fighting not for territory but for values.

The implication is that the distinction between humanitarian aid and humanitarian intervention is disappearing. Of course military and humanitarian action is not the same. Bombing Kosovo is not equivalent to providing food and shelter to Kosovar refugees. But both are becoming more and more interdependent. Military interventions are legitimised by calling on humanitarian organisations; these organisations need the military to guarantee their safety. More importantly, both have the same aim: rescuing the innocent and helpless. Both are guided by the same sentiments of compassion and humanity. Both appeal to a higher moral order (Wheeler 1997). Conflicts and disasters are now included in the same logic of humanitarian relief (Fassin and Pandolfi 2010). This contemporary logic reflects an important change in international thinking due to processes of globalisation. The principle of non-intervention that used to regulate the relations between nations was based on the value of national sovereignty and on the position that states only act when it is in their own interest and not for moral reasons. This respect for state sovereignty is now superseded by the global norms of human rights and human dignity. National sovereignty has a subsidiary value. It is therefore conditional: states only have immunity from foreign intervention as long as they treat their citizens decently. In other words, the political order is now subordinated in a global moral order. States are subject to a higher normative order. The underlying conception is that of global moral community or shared humanity (Nardin 2009). The same process is at work in the expansion of bioethics into global bioethics. The notion of moral community is extended to the global level. At this level universal principles are at work, which request us to prevent or mitigate evil when we have the capacity to do so. The ultimate sovereign of the global community is humanity, one of the defining principles of humanitarian action (Charvet 1997). The moral imperative to assist and intervene is expressed in a new language of humanitarianism, emphasising cosmopolitanism, common humanity and the responsibility to protect (R2P) and focusing on the victim's point of view (Benhabib 2009).

2.3.3 Emergency Ethics

The war in Biafra (1967–1970) was the origin of the so-called second phase of modern humanitarianism. Because the Nigerian government did not allow any relief into the area where it was most needed, some Red Cross doctors departed from the principle of neutrality and spoke out for the victims. This led to the establishment of the new relief organisation Médecins sans Frontières (MSF) in 1971. The Red Cross has been criticised for its consistent stance of impartiality and neutrality, for example, when it visited the Nazi concentration camps during World War II but did not report on what was going on there, or more recently when Red Cross workers paid visits to Guantanamo Bay only on condition that they did not report (Brauman 2009). The basic idea of MSF is that in some circumstances it might be in the interest of the victims not to maintain silence but to speak out. One cannot close one's eyes to violations of human rights, especially when the parties that are committing those violations are also in control of the relief efforts. Not taking sides and remaining silent is no longer in the interests of the victims; in such conditions one has to testify about the injustices and violations. Intervention may be mandated, in the words of Bernard Kouchner, by an 'emergency ethics' ('une morale de l'extrême urgence'; Perrot 2006).

The foundation of MSF symbolises the change from aid to action. It represents an ethics in action, promoting humanitarianism as a new repertoire for public action (Fassin 2007). For many people today, humanitarianism is synonymous with 'doing good'; it is the symbol of selfless action; it represents the ideal of a better, more humane world (Barnett and Weiss 2008). The prototype of the humanitarian worker is the Good Samaritan. The moral reasoning behind humanitarian action is obvious: protect populations, save lives, relieve suffering.

However, the humanitarian discourse cannot be taken for granted. It incorporates and expresses particular values that are taken as self-evident but often these values are given priority over other possible values. It is also assumed that emergencies, exceptions and the need to intervene are self-evident, as if we would not have other choices from an ethical perspective. In this regard it is interesting to study the work of the French physician and anthropologist Didier Fassin who has analysed the humanitarian discourse (Fassin 2007, 2008, 2010).

The fundamental value of this discourse is human life. The basic justification of humanitarian action is saving life. This is the first-order principle, while neutrality, impartiality or consent are second-order principles. This principle inspires the world view of many nongovernmental organisations (NGOs): they come in to assist vulnerable populations, to help victims of natural or man-made disasters. They have no political agenda or power claims. Their only power consists in the powerless. In distinction to politics which sacrifices, humanitarianism saves and rescues. In the fight between good and evil, they are on the right side.

Humanitarianism is also a powerful discourse since it combines the rational and the emotional. Humanitarian reason is inspiring solidarity, and humanitarian sentiment motivates compassion. These two dimensions are embedded in the notion 'humanitas' (the French term 'humanité' has the same double meaning): humanity as an ethical category including all human beings ('humankind', 'Menschheit') is the basis for solidarity; and humanity as concern for other human beings ('humaneness'; 'Menschlichkeit') is the basis for compassion, even with distant suffering. The bringing together of solidarity and compassion implies that there should not be distinctions among human beings (humanity is one and indivisible) nor should there be indifference to distant others. Distance and distinction are simultaneously transcended in the same discourse.

Fassin shows that in humanitarian practice things are more complicated. Human lives are not equal. There is always a balance between lives to be saved and lives to be risked. When a Stanford emergency team arrived in Haiti 5 days after the earthquake in 2010, they provided care to hundreds of people in the university hospital. But at the end of the day the medical team was leaving the hospital (because of security reasons) knowing that nobody was available to manage the pain and take care of patients during the night (Camacho-McAdoo 2010). Humanitarian missions can be dangerous. Although biologically, lives are the same, philosophically they are different. Humanitarian workers can choose to sacrifice themselves for a good cause. Victims have no choice, they are sacrificed (in the language of Fassin). Because lives are sacred, humanitarianism can demand the potential sacrifice of one's life. But there is a difference between 'bare life' to be assisted and the political life that is freely risked, or between the *zoe* of populations harmed by disasters and the *bios* of citizens of the world who come to their rescue (Agamben 1998). Not all lives have the same value. Fassin (2007) demonstrates this with the example of policies in case aid workers are kidnapped or abducted, and with the difference made in MSF missions between expatriate and national staff. The same inequality pertains in humanitarian interventions. For the sacred life of the intervening 'humanitarian' soldier, it is deemed worth sacrificing the life of hundreds or thousands of people (soldiers or not) on the other side.

Humanitarianism therefore should be defined as "politics of life" (Fassin 2007). It is different from the 'biopolitics' espoused by Michel Foucault since it is not concerned about populations but rather with the lives of individuals. At the same time it is politics since it implies selecting which lives are possibly or legitimately to be saved. For example, humanitarian workers have to consider which AIDS patients should receive antiretroviral medications, or whether assistance should be provided to persons who have participated in massacres.

The radical inequality of lives is furthermore demonstrated in the creation of victimhood (Fassin and Rechtman 2009). The articulation of reason and emotion in humanitarianism is generating a specific attitude towards other human beings. The other is regarded as vulnerable and traumatised. He or she no longer is a survivor or hero but a victim (Debrix 1998). In his studies of the Palestinian Territories, Fassin shows how humanitarianism translates political domination and violence into suffering and trauma. The focus on human life transforms people who are resisting or protesting into victims. Humanitarianism requires protecting and caring for all victims; there are neither good nor bad victims. But one can never help all victims. Tragic choices need to be made.

Contemporary humanitarianism as ethics in action is not only providing care but also bearing witness. It is speaking out on behalf of the victims. Such humanitarian testimony introduces a distinction between those who are subject (the witnesses who testify, usually the humanitarian workers) and those who are object (the victims whose suffering is testified). Those who show compassion take on the role of witness for those they assist. Testimony in this way reiterates two forms of humanity: those who can tell stories and those whose stories can only be told by others. Again 'bare life' is transformed into qualified 'political life'. Through the humanitarian testimony mere physical survival will become social existence that is more powerful in eliciting compassion and the need for assistance. But the transforming act is done by a third person, the transforming subject, i.e. the humanitarian worker. At the same time the object of transformation is reduced to victim. The young Palestinian stone thrower is no longer a hero but has become fragile, vulnerable, traumatised. The logic of compassion is replacing the demand for justice (Fassin 2008).

2.4 Different Perspectives

Humanitarianism as politics of life is nowadays the most powerful language for public action. It is re-establishing solidarity among human beings and it gives equal value to all lives. Humanitarianism is furthermore the best contemporary expression of a cosmopolitan ethics in which international borders, cultural diversities and political ideologies are irrelevant in the face of human suffering. But in practice it is problematic since it not merely highlights the value of human life but is also associated with, in the words of Fassin, a 'complex ontology of inequality' (Fassin 2007, p. 219). It makes distinctions between lives that may be risked and lives that can be sacrificed, between lives that have higher value and those that have limited protection, and between lives that are narrated in the first person and lives that are only recounted in the third person. Finally it is problematic as politics since it is introducing morality into the political sphere. Fassin does not hesitate to speak of a new type of governance, *viz.* 'humanitarian government' (Fassin and Pandolfi 2010). Now that political ideology has retreated since the end of the Cold War, the space is filled by humanitarianism which is now the apogee of the ideal of human solidarity. The new discourse demands that we assist, even if necessary intervene, because it is a moral obligation rather than a legal or political principle. The politics of assistance and intervention are now justified in the name of humanitarian morality. Protection of peoples and saving lives is more important than respect for the sovereignty of states. Morality justifies the suspension of the rule of law. The ethics of emergency presupposes that we live in a state of exception established at global level. There are perennial emergencies. Nothing is normal. The continuous state of exception is justified by the urgency of situations (emergencies) as well as the danger to the victims (rescue, protection, security).

The same logic of intervention can therefore be applied in assisting the victims of civil war in Somalia as in aiding the victims of the tsunami in Sri Lanka. The paradigm of disaster prevails over the paradigm of war. In this logic there is no essential difference between disasters and conflicts. The world's disorders, whether natural or human in origin, become humanised. Natural disasters become humanised—not simply the result of brute force of nature; while violence and conflict become naturalised—not merely the result of brute human force. By equating the two types of emergencies, the only issue is aid to the victims; the local context with its history and socio-economic tensions is less relevant. Human conflicts become depoliticised: the historical background and the conflict setting are displaced by urgency and compassion. But it also means that macro-ethical questions regarding disasters are no longer relevant.

2.4.1 The Value of Life and Justice

At the same time, solidarity and compassion are not unlimited. Humanitarian efforts cannot relieve all suffering everywhere. And interventions to bring about a world in which violations of human dignity do not take place are a drop in the ocean. Often humanitarianism is selective (Brown 2003). We intervene in Libya but not in Yemen, Bahrain or Syria. There are also huge gaps in aid spending: $33.9 million per death from Hurricane Katrina in 2005, $35,336 per death from the 2004 tsunami, $2,483 per death in the 2005 Pakistan earthquake, and $1,968 per HIV/AIDS death in 2004 (Wolinsky 2007). Similar differences exist in famine aid. Substantially more food aid was generated for Kosovar refugees in 1998 than for Liberian refugees in the same period of time (Rinehart 2002). If all human lives are of equal value, why is there unequal treatment?

Elaborating on the differences in responses to large-scale human tragedies like the 2004 tsunami and the HIV/AIDS pandemic, Christie et al. (2007) suggest that it might be the apparent morally neutral nature of the tsunami disaster that was responsible for the massive resource mobilisation. Nobody is to blame for a natural disaster, and the victims are clearly innocent, while HIV/AIDS is spread via human conduct. This different response illustrates once again the inequality of human life that is associated with humanitarianism. It also illustrates the powerful rhetoric of disasters as natural events that can drive public generosity and the philanthropic enterprise. The international response to the catastrophe is ethically praiseworthy but should at the same time be ethically criticised since it is unjust. There is no morally relevant difference between the two tragedies justifying the difference in response. The discrepancy makes clear that human life is not the only relevant value at stake; justice is another.

2.4.2 *Triaging Humanitarian Interventions*

The critique of selective humanitarianism has instigated reflection on the moral criteria for choosing where and when to relieve suffering. Brown (2003) for example has suggested simple triage rules for deciding what sorts of interventions should be undertaken. He distinguishes three categories of situations in the world: (1) difficulties that are sufficiently minor that intervention would do more harm than good, (2) difficulties that are of such magnitude that action would be ineffective (e.g. the devastation is simply too extensive, like in the Democratic Republic of Congo) or would be counterproductive (e.g. in Tibet or Chechnya where a powerful government can make intervention into a more widespread disaster), and (3) situations where intervention is practically possible and has the prospect of bringing improvements. In developing selection criteria many political philosophers in fact are taking older criteria from the Just War tradition (just cause; right intention; proper authority; proportionality; last resort; prospect of success; care being taken to protect the innocent) and applying them to the circumstances of humanitarian intervention (Coady 2003).

2.4.3 *Allocation Decisions in Aid*

How are resource allocation decisions made in humanitarian aid? Some commentators are pessimistic and accept that there is no rational coordination, no commonly shared targets, and no clear rationale; there is just ‘chaotic do-gooder-ism’ (Wolinsky 2007). Often decision-making is not transparent. Most NGOs are self-mandating and self-regulating; they have full discretionary power over what they do. Fuller (2006) examined the justifications given for resource allocation decisions at Headquarters level in MSF and identified three types:

1. Public health perspective. Decisions are based on population statistics (e.g., the outbreak of specific diseases). As soon as the outbreak is controlled, it is useful to close a project; the disaster is over. This type of decision-making is most appropriate in an acute crisis focused on a particular problem. The most urgent need has priority.

2. Organisational perspective. Decisions are based on the mandate or mission of the organisation. For MSF for example, there should be a crisis with humanitarian and medical components.
3. Community perspective. Decisions are based on advocacy arguments. Relationships already exist between certain populations, and these relationships generate special responsibilities. The projects are also setting an example; they show that certain treatments will work in certain circumstances.

Instead of identifying a set of clear criteria, Fuller's study reveals competing moral views. Those views are focused on the one hand on severity of need and the likelihood of securing good outcomes or on the urgency of the situation. On the other hand they are focused on the existing relationships of trust, cooperation, vulnerability and dependence. All views presuppose the basic value of saving human lives but differences appear in connection with the means to accomplish the goals of rescue and protection. It is clear that a comprehensive framework of selection criteria is lacking, although some elements reminiscent of the Just War theory are there, such as considerations of cause, means and ends (Ford et al. 2010).

2.4.4 Human Life and Human Rights

Even if today's humanitarianism is considered as emergency ethics, many humanitarian efforts are in fact struggling with more values than simply saving human lives (Slim 1997). The value of life continuously competes with values like human dignity and justice. As mentioned earlier, the focus on human life transforms people into victims. This will position them as traumatised persons in need, putting the social and political context between brackets. Humanitarianism as politics of life will also continuously evoke our sentiments of compassion. By calling for philanthropy, generosity and charity it will never basically challenge the politics that permit war, famine and suffering. The ethical drive embedded in humanitarianism is so strong and compelling that it can hardly be criticised; at the same time, it directs our focus on immediate relief for individual victims so that we tend to forget that other dimensions are equally important. One dimension, mentioned above, is the social context which is often unjust. Another dimension is the perspective of the recipient. In many humanitarian operations the persons who receive assistance are absent and silent (Barnett and Weiss 2008). The failure to give voice to the vulnerable is remarkable since the ethics of humanitarianism is based on the notion of human dignity.

It is therefore argued that humanitarianism should be redefined in terms of rights (Slim 2002). Instead of the language of needs and compassion we should use the language of human rights and dignity. Within the recent discourses of the United Nations, the Red Cross and NGOs, more emphasis is needed nowadays on rights-based humanitarianism. Poverty and development have been redefined in terms of human rights.

The advantage of this approach is that humanitarianism will be grounded on an integrated moral-legal framework of international human rights law. It will be more than just a moral endeavour but will also be anchored in institutions (courts, tribunals, truth commissions), even if they are not recognised by all states.

The second advantage is that rights dignify rather than victimise. People are no longer regarded as needy victims but as citizens of the world with the same claims and rights as everyone else. Human rights make people equal and more powerful. They provide a universal and objective standard to assess human behaviour (Slim 2002). This does not ignore the many problems in the global application of this approach. But the fact is that all states have and still are participating in the norm-creating process in which these international standards are articulated.

The third advantage of the human rights approach is that it generates foreign policy imperatives as expressions of international responsibility. Membership of the international community entails recognition of the moral urgency of human rights. Kelly (2004) has identified three such moral obligations: non-engagement, aid, and intervention. The modalities of humanitarianism are, in his view, guided by the shared concern for human rights.

2.5 Conclusion

Analysing disaster planning and humanitarian aid from a macro-ethical perspective produces a paradoxical conclusion: macro-issues concerning context and background are irrelevant in the prevailing logic of disaster relief. What ethically matters in today's humanitarianism is saving lives, rescuing individuals and protecting populations.

The dominant ethical framework of disaster relief has two consequences. First, the focus on emergency ethics makes it difficult to provide structural, long-term aid. Global intervention and assistance are driven by compassion with fellow human beings in situations of crisis. But why does this recognition of our common humanity not lead us to consider deeper causes of suffering in the social and economic context? We feel compelled to act as moral agents out of solidarity with the global community but then we only address crises and emergencies, not the human wrongs of poverty and starvation. It seems that we don't spare efforts to save the lives of victims of sudden natural disasters but accept the slow death through poverty and malnutrition. The public health system around the globe has more or less collapsed (Garrett 2007). Poor living conditions in many countries are the source of global disease threats. Even the efficiency of humanitarian aid is rather low if poor hygiene and sanitary conditions will not be improved. While each day more than 10,000 children die from diarrhoea, suffering only seems to generate compassion and humanitarian relief if it is caused by natural disasters. This focus of humanitarian assistance can easily be regarded as an alibi for not changing lifestyle and consumption patterns in countries providing such assistance (Wheeler 1997). Despite all the compassion, charity and solidarity, global suffering continues. We have not learned the lessons from an earlier decade when bioterrorism was presented as a major threat to health and security. Since the 1990s tens of billions have been spent on 'biodefense' (King 2005). Preparedness programs have created the impression of immediate action. But in fact resources have been spent for hypothetical threats and were diverted away from more pressing public health needs.

The second consequence of humanitarian emergency ethics is that the voice of the recipient of assistance is absent. Again an analogy can be made with the approach of homeland security in the United States. A massive security apparatus and bureaucracy has been established that enforces top-down security measures. Civil society and citizens are not engaged. Individual resilience is not promoted so that in fact individuals have become increasingly complacent and helpless in the face of threats and disasters (Flynn 2011). In the perspective of humanitarian aid, the distant others who are harmed by disasters are helpless and vulnerable; they deserve compassion and assistance. In reality, most survivors of disasters owe their lives to neighbours and local authorities. It is a myth that they are waiting to be saved by international rescue teams (De Ville de Goyet 2000). Nonetheless, the relationship between provider and recipient of assistance is often asymmetrical. The recipients are not the ones that determine their own needs. They are not visible as moral agents but as devastated, silent victims. With the best intentions aid is provided but often with a reduced view of the person as only being in need of basic issues such as food, water, shelter and medical care. Recipients are not supposed to participate in determining their own destiny. Brauman (2009) illustrates how this may lead to misdirected aid. During the war in Mogadishu for example the only way to save the life of some persons was by amputation. But many wounded young people refused to be amputated since they did want to live with a visible mutilation. During the recent Haiti earthquake several thousand people were amputated without consideration of their long-term quality of life in one of the poorest nations in the world. What is beneficial for the disaster victim can only be determined through focusing on the larger context of human reality beyond the immediate emergency situation. Within the perspective of emergency ethics what counts is saving the life of the victim but what is forgotten is life before and after victimhood.

References

Agamben, Giorgio. 1998. *Homo sacer. Sovereign power and bare life*. Stanford: Stanford University Press.

ACEP (American College of Emergency Physicians). 2011. Advancing emergency care: Policy compendium. http://www.acep.org/policystatements/. Accessed 1 May 2013.

Barnett, Michael, and Thomas G. Weiss. 2008. Humanitarianism. A brief history of the present. In *Humanitarianism in question. Politics, power, ethics,* eds. Michael Barnett and Thomas G. Weiss, 1–48. Ithaca: Cornell University Press.

Barnett, D. J., H. A. Taylor, J. G. Hodge, and J. M. Links. 2009. Resource allocation on the frontlines of public health preparedness and response: Report of a summit on legal and ethical issues. *Public Health Reports* 124:295–303.

Benhabib, Sheyla. 2009. On the alleged conflict between democracy and international law. In *Ethics & International Affairs. A reader,* eds. Joel H. Rosenthal, and Christian Barry, 185–203. Washington D.C.: Georgetown University Press.

Berg, Jessica, and Nancy King. 2006. Strange bedfellows? Reflections on bioethics' role in disaster response planning. *American Journal of Bioethics* 6 (5): 3–5.

Brauman, Rony. 2009. *La médicine humanitaire*. Paris: Presses Universitaires de France.

Brown, Chris. 2003. Selective humanitarianism: In defense of inconsistency. In *Ethics and foreign intervention,* eds. Deen K. Chatterdjee and Don E. Scheid, 31–50. Cambridge: Cambridge University Press.

Camacho-McAdoo, G. 2010. Triage following a natural disaster: A haitian experience. *Journal of Emergency Nursing* 36:385–387.

Charvet, J. 1997. The idea of state sovereignty and the right of humanitarian intervention. *International Political Science Review* 18 (1): 39–48.

Chatterdjee, Deen K., and Don E. Scheid. 2003. *Ethics and foreign intervention.* Cambridge: Cambridge University Press.

Christie, T., G. A. Asrat, B. Jiwani, T. Maddix, and J.S.G. Montaner. 2007. Exploring disparities between global HIV/AIDS funding and recent tsunami relief efforts: An ethical analysis. *Developing World Bioethics* 7 (1): 1–7.

Clark, N. 2005. Disaster and generosity. *The Geographical Journal* 171:384–386.

Coady, C. A. J. 2003. War for humanity: A critique. In *Ethics and foreign intervention,* eds. Deen K. Chatterdjee and Don E. Scheid, 274–295. Cambridge: Cambridge University Press.

Debrix, F. 1998. Deterritorialised territories, borderless borders: The new geography of international medical assistance. *Third World Quarterly* 19 (5): 827–846.

De Ville de Goyet, C. 2000. Stop propagating disaster myths. *Lancet* 356:762–764.

Etienne, M., C. Powell, and D. Amundson. 2010. Healthcare ethics: The experience after the Haitian earthquake. *American Journal of Disaster Medicine* 5 (3): 141–147.

Fassin, Didier. 2007. Humanitarianism as a politics of life. *Public Culture* 19 (3): 499–520.

Fassin, Didier. 2008. The humanitarian politics of testimony. Subjectification through trauma in the Israeli-Palestinian conflict. *Cultural Anthropology* 23 (3): 531–558.

Fassin, Didier. 2010. Heart of humaneness: The moral economy of humanitarian intervention. In *Contemporary states of emergency. The politics of military and humanitarian interventions,* eds. Fassin Didier and Pandolfi Mariella, 269–293. New York: Zone Books.

Fassin, Didier, and Mariella Pandolfi, eds. 2010. *Contemporary states of emergency. The politics of military and humanitarian interventions*. New York: Zone Books.

Fassin, Didier, and Richard Rechtman. 2009. *The empire of trauma. An inquiry into the condition of victimhood.* Princeton: Princeton University Press.

Flynn, S. 2011. Recalibrating homeland security. Mobilizing American society to prepare for disaster. *Foreign Affairs* 90 (3): 130–140.

Ford, N., R. Zachariah, E. Mills, and R. Upshur. 2010. Defining the limits of emergency humanitarian action: Where, and how, to draw the line? *Public Health Ethics* 3 (1): 68–71.

Fuller, L. 2006. Justified commitments? Considering resource allocation and fairness in Médecins Sans Frontières—Holland. *Developing World Bioethics* 6 (2): 59–70.

Garrett, L. 2007. The challenge of global health. *Foreign Affairs* 86 (1): 14–38.

Hattori, T. 2003. The moral politics of foreign aid. *Review of International Studies* 29:229–247.

Herkert, J. R. 2001. Future directions in engineering ethics research: Microethics, macroethics and the role of professional societies. *Science and Engineering Ethics* 7:403–414.

Hodge, J. G. 2006. Legal triage during public health emergencies and disasters. *Administrative Law Review* 58:627–644.

International Federation of Red Cross and Red Crescent Societies. 2010. *World Disaster Report*. Geneva. http://www.ifrc.org/Global/Publications/disasters/WDR/WDR2010-full.pdf. Accessed 4 June 2013.

Kelly, Erin. 2004. Human rights as foreign policy imperatives. In *The ethics of assistance. Morality and the distant needy,* ed. Deen K. Chatterdjee, 177–192. Cambridge: Cambridge University Press.

King, N.B. 2005. The ethics of biodefense. *Bioethics* 19 (4): 432–446.

Korf, B. 2006. Disasters, generosity and the other. *The Geographical Journal* 172:245–247.

Lakoff, Andrew. 2007. Preparing for the next emergency. *Public Culture* 19 (2): 247–271.

Lakoff, Andrew. 2008. The generic biothreat, or, how we became unprepared. *Cultural Anthropology* 23 (3): 399–428.

Lin, Y.A., and L. Anderson-Shaw. 2009. Rationing of resources: Ethical issues in disasters and epidemic situations. *Prehospital and Disaster Medicine* 24 (3): 215–221.

Macintyre, B. 2010. The fault line in Haiti runs straight to France. The Times, January 21. http://www.timesonline.co.uk/tol/comment/columnists/ben_macintyre/article6995750.ece. Accessed 4 June 2013.

Middleton, Neil. 2010. *Humanitarian assistance? Haiti and beyond.* London: Seagull Books.

Nardin, Terry. 2009. The moral basis of humanitarian intervention. In *Ethics & international affairs. A reader,* eds. Joel H. Rosenthal and Christian Barry, 85–101. Washington, DC: Georgetown University Press.

NATO. 2011. *Emergency war surgery*. Seattle: Pacific Publishing Studio.

Newberry, B. 2010. Katrina: Macro-ethical issues for engineers. *Science and Engineering Ethics* 16:535–571.

Pellegrino, Edmund D. 1976. Philosophy of medicine: Problematic and potential. *Journal of Medicine and Philosophy* 1 (1): 5–31.

Perrot, S. 2006. Devoir et droit d'ingérence. Réseau francophone de recherche sur les operations de paix. http://gervaisdjidji.over-blog.fr/article-devoir-et-droit-d-ingerence-65614086.html. Accessed 4 June 2013.

Petrini, C. 2010. Triage in public health emergencies: Ethical issues. *Internal and Emergency Medicine* 5:137–144.

Rinehart, A. 2002. Famine relief: Just a simple matter of supplying food? *Nutrition Noteworthy* 5 (1): 1–7. http://escholarship.org/uc/item/81×2g9z2;jsessionid=49A643C1F88BF69CCDA1D407779A88B9. Accessed 4 June 2013.

Slim, H. 1997. Doing the right thing: Relief agencies, moral dilemmas and moral responsibility in political emergencies and war. *Disasters* 21 (3): 244–257.

Slim, H. 2002. Not philanthropy but rights: The proper politicisation of humanitarian philosophy. *The International Journal of Human Rights* 6 (2): 1–22.

Smith, Michael J. 2009. Humanitarian intervention. An overview of the ethical issues. In *Ethics & international affairs. A reader,* eds. Joel H. Rosenthal and Christian Barry, 67–83. Washington, DC: Georgetown University Press.

Son, W. 2008. Philosophy of technology and macro-ethics in engineering. *Science and Engineering Ethics* 14:405–415.

Sztajnkrycer, M.D., B. E. Madsen, and A. A. Baez. 2006. Unstable ethical plateaus and disaster triage. *Emergency Medicine Clinics of North America* 24:749–768.

Ten Have, Henk. 2004. Ethical perspective on health technology assessment. *International Journal of Technology Assessment in Health Care* 20 (1): 71–76.

Walzer, Michael. 1995. The politics and rescue. *Social Research* 62 (1): 53–66.

Wheeler, N.J. 1997. Agency, humanitarianism and intervention. *International Political Science Review* 18 (1): 9–25.

Wikipedia. 2011 http://en.wikipedia.org/wiki/List_of_settlements_lost_to_floods_in_the_Netherlands. Accessed 16 Mar 2011.

Wolinsky, H. 2007. Bioethics goes global. *EMBO Reports* 8 (6): 534–536.

Chapter 3
Ethics and Emergency Disaster Response. Normative Approaches and Training Needs for Humanitarian Health Care Providers

Lisa Schwartz, Matthew Hunt, Lynda Redwood-Campbell and Sonya de Laat

3.1 History of the Project

The study grew out of personal experiences of some of the co-investigators who had been part of emergency responses after disasters such as the 2004 tsunami and the 2005 earthquake in Pakistan, and on development missions in Eastern Europe, Africa and Asia. As our interest in the topic grew, we heard more and more anecdotal evidence of ethical challenges experienced by health care providers in humanitarian health care, and began to recognise the need for applied ethical theory in humanitarian health care practice.

In North America, when health care providers encounter ethical challenges they have a variety of resources available to draw from. They have codes of professional practice, acknowledged ethical frameworks and a conceptual vocabulary for describing ethical issues. In most hospitals, there are ethics committees or ethics consultants to help avoid and resolve conflicts and improve outcomes for patients, families and practitioners (Fox et al. 2007; DuVal et al. 2001).

In acute disaster response, there are few, if any, such resources. Some scant examples exist of formal ethics interventions during field missions such as the Israeli field hospital and US Navy in Haiti (Merin 2010; Etienne 2010), but these are sparse and case specific. Not surprisingly, given media fascination with scandal, there are far more published examples of questionable or unethical activities (Costello 2012; Sontag 2010). Very few empirically informed resources guide ethical practice in humanitarian health care.

L. Schwartz (✉)
McMaster University, Hamilton, Canada
e-mail: schwar@mcmaster.ca

M. Hunt
McGill University, Montreal, Canada

L. Redwood-Campbell · S. de Laat
McMaster University, Hamilton, Canada

D. P. O'Mathúna et al. (eds.), *Disaster Bioethics: Normative Issues When Nothing is Normal,* Public Health Ethics Analysis 2, DOI 10.1007/978-94-007-3864-5_3,

On the strength of the anecdotal evidence and preliminary exploration of existing literature and resources in humanitarian health care ethics, we formed a research team and began the study, *Ethics in conditions of disaster and deprivation: Learning from health workers' narratives*.[1] The team is multi-disciplinary, consisting of academics from philosophy and ethics, social sciences, anthropology, and clinicians from nursing, physiotherapy, a surgical oncologist and a public health trained family doctor. We drew on grounded theory to inform the qualitative study of in-depth interviews with 20 humanitarian health care professionals who had travelled with aid organisations or independently in response to disaster, poverty or conflict. The respondents included nurses, nurse practitioners, physicians, physiotherapists, lab specialists and public health practitioners. They had travelled to Africa, Asia, South America and the Caribbean on an average of four missions each, with a range of 1–12 (Schwartz et al. 2010).

3.2 Results of the Study

Analysis of the stories revealed four broad sources of ethical challenges for humanitarian health care providers (Schwartz et al. 2010). The most frequent causes of ethical challenge reported by the respondents are briefly described here. Anonymous quotations come from respondent interviews.

3.2.1 The Four Themes

a. Resource scarcity: Tension arose between knowing you can only do so much, perceiving much more was needed, and wanting deeply to do more (Sinding et al. 2010).

   > I have no resources, I can't see everybody. I'm not providing optimal care you know. We tried wherever possible.

b. Inequalities associated with historical, political, social and commercial structures: participants struggled to figure out how to respect local norms and sustain their own values; they also worried about the lingering impact of previous injustice such as colonial histories.

   > Whether our aid is truly helping or whether we are in enabling a toxic situation in the sense that we are providing free healthcare for migrant workers and migrant workers who work on commercial farms ... But certainly we question if we are directly assisting a for-profit industry.

c. Aid agency policies and agendas: directives from aid agencies, such as security directives and vertical programing, sometimes conflicted with what respondents understood to be their professional or ethical duties.

---

[1] The study received funding from the Canadian Institutes of Health Research (CIHR) Ethics Office in 2008, and research ethics approval from the McMaster University Faculty of Health Sciences Research Ethics Board.

> It made me feel a little cruel because here we show up with our Land Cruiser with the flag flying, we come whisking in and I'm sure that that healthcare provider took an exhale. Great help has arrived, we can do this together. And then to see me come in with my clipboard and you know do a few calculations and then wave good bye and drive away must have just been ...

d. Professional norms: differences in resources and cultural understandings of illness created misunderstandings; professional hierarchies and cultural differences were sometimes thorny and complicated decision-making.

> And patients I mean that is the way it is so obviously the physician's word is what is taken ... So I could never say to the physician 'I think you are wrong'.

In addition, as a cross-cutting theme, the collected stories demonstrated the consequences of ethical struggles, uncertainty and conflict for the personal and professional identities of the respondents. As described elsewhere (Schwartz et al. 2010), actions that participants felt were intrinsic to 'being a nurse' or 'being a doctor' or 'being a physiotherapist' could not always be enacted because of crisis settings, scarce resources, or because of a social or cultural norm, the political situation or policy directives.

> I felt all of a sudden as if I was not a nurse anymore. I was just me and I was just looking at something and I had no way of doing anything about it.

The stories told by the respondents indicated that ethical challenges arose for multiple reasons. The cases were always complex, so more than one of the causes arose simultaneously. Due to the frequency and challenging nature of the ethical issues reported by the study participants, and the understanding that they are not unique, it is essential that aid workers be supported to address the ethical issues they encounter while providing health care in disaster settings. Inability to provide what they perceive to be adequate care leads to stress and burn-out of healthcare professionals (Schwartz et al. 2010). Humanitarian healthcare providers need training in managing ethical conflicts. Some resources do exist to guide ethical action in the field and new ones are emerging. We propose that careful consideration be given to which resources can most usefully be employed.

The study we draw from included health care professionals involved in many different kinds of humanitarian response, so it is broader than disaster. Nevertheless, the themes are relevant to disaster responders and we will focus on this context for the remainder of the chapter.

3.3 Mapping the Existing Landscape

Health care professionals who participate in disaster relief response are trained in clinical ethics derived from their home contexts. These ethics approaches tend to be individual patient oriented and presuppose comparatively well-resourced settings in places such as Canada, Europe, and the United States. While similar categories describe ethical issues in these countries, the quality of the experience in disasters is certainly different: resources are not merely scarce but can be non-existent; practices, such as triage, may be managed differently; in disasters, systems are in crisis and supports may be strained to the limit; in addition, needs are more extreme and more numerous. Respondents frequently drew comparisons to their home contexts,

> I don't know because it's also very hard when I think of some of these clinical ethical issues that I've spoken about like a preemie or whatnot. It's hard because I know sometimes here we tend to say 'well in Canada . . . ' and I just realize in Canada it's so different from in Haiti and I appreciate that the doctors and nurses kind of would just roll their eyes and be like 'well this is Haiti' or whatever. So I guess I don't know how relevant any of what we were taught would be . . .

In contrast, the demands associated with disaster situations are not individually oriented but tend to compel a 'greater good' focus. In disaster response, for example, there are overriding concerns about infection control among the affected population; prevention of cholera is one case in point. The context, therefore, sometimes blurs clear distinctions between the perspective of public health practice and the perspective of clinical health practice. As a result, humanitarian health care ethics may be better guided by the values of both clinical and public health ethics together (Schwartz et al. 2012).

However, of the twenty respondents interviewed in our study, only two had public health training prior to their first missions. Notably, three were inspired by their field experience to pursue public health certification later on. For the most part, the respondents entered the field with intentions of doing the best they could with the skills and knowledge they had gained as health care professionals in clinical settings within their home countries. Tensions then emerged because of the difference in focus, loyalties and the demands of clinical as opposed to public health practice. This divided their attention between individual best interest of a particular patient and the wider interests of the affected community.

Another difference is in the way triage is managed. In well-resourced, home settings, healthcare practitioners are trained that triage is based on the assumption that all will eventually receive treatment, which means it is possible to prioritise those who are in greatest need and likely to die. In a disaster setting, where resources are strained and needs are numerous, it is likely that decisions to treat will be focused on those who are most likely to benefit from the treatment. Patients whose deaths appear imminent may be left untreated, sometimes without even comfort measures or palliation.

The respondents struggled to justify what they perceived to be calculated and unavoidable injustices where the genuine needs of individual patients could not be attended to due to contextual exigencies. These tensions are not easily managed, and may well be inevitable (de Waal 2010), but the ethical tensions were surely aggravated by the respondents' feelings that they were ill-prepared to handle them.

3.4 Professional Codes

In some cases, organisations rely on codes of ethics of regulatory bodies in the responders' home countries to provide ethical guidance.

> Médecins Sans Frontières' volunteers promise to honour their professional code of ethics . . . (Médecins Sans Frontiéres 2013)

These codes are undoubtedly excellent foundational guidance for health care practitioners in the field. However, they are not designed to provide guidance in extreme settings such as disaster, nor are they necessarily consistent with host country norms and expectations, so they may be insufficient on their own. More consideration should be given to the establishment of international codes of ethics, such as the World Medical Association (WMA 2006) international code for disaster response. International codes, created in dialogue with countries that have received aid in disaster conditions, will make the codes better informed and more responsive to the extreme conditions of disaster settings.

The following case is based on the experience of one of the authors and reflects situations recounted by our study participants. It illustrates how policies and mission remits have ethical impact because they confound the ethical priorities issued by western models of professional clinical ethics.

3.5 Case 1: After the Waters Came

After a particular natural disaster, a field hospital was established with a mandate to treat disaster-related surgical cases only. Nine weeks later, 88 % of the patients at the field hospital presented with health problems that were not directly related. Due to a lack of local resources and clinical staff (80 % of local health facilities were either destroyed or non-functional), these patients had few alternatives and could not rely on the local healthcare system (Redwood-Campbell and Riddez 2006).

A man about 35 years old came to the unit with a massive inguinal hernia. He described how this was affecting his livelihood as a farmer, and that it limited his ability to support his already impoverished family. A surgeon who had the skills to repair the patient's hernia asked for permission to treat him even though his hernia was a long-standing condition that had been present prior to the disaster (the farmer had no financial means of paying for the surgery in any case). It was decided by management that it was outside of the hospital's mandate to do this type of elective procedure.

The unit manager forwarded this request to the aid agency's head office in Europe, which refused to grant permission for the surgery because it was outside the field hospital's mandate. In spite of this mandate, and a clear directive to abide by it, the team struggled to decide whether they should provide elective surgery in this situation.

The case outlines some important issues for ethical humanitarian health care practice. First the aid agency had an agreement with the local government to provide emergency response care and had an obligation to respect the parameters of that agreement. Similarly, aid organisations rely on charitable donations and have an ethical obligation to respect the wishes of their donors who donate funds for specific responses, or clarify to the donors that the funds may be used for other purposes. So the aid agency restrictions required the field hospital staff to act within certain limitations as a matter of policy and to protect the aid agency's wider agenda to provide aid.

Resource limitation was an additional factor. Aid agencies do not have endless resources and need to allocate what they do have in a fair manner. In this case, there were so many legitimate and pressing health needs within the population that restrictions had to be set otherwise the resources might not be available for the people for whom they were intended. On the other hand, clinicians were confronted with the health need of a specific individual. They were trained to respond to this need, and saw it as their duty to do so. In ideal circumstances all needs would be met, but the circumstances after a disaster are far from ideal and in this case alternate access to health care was vanishingly limited. An ethical challenge was created from the circumstances of scarce resources, genuine need, the consequences of (not) treating and the obligations of the health professionals to the patient as opposed to those of the aid agency to the government and donors.

Beyond the multiple obligations, prioritising was out of the hands of the clinicians in the field hospital who were expected to follow aid agency protocols and policies. The result was a conflict of needs, loyalties and duties. It is a complex case, made all the more challenging by the circumstances of disaster, multiple obligations and international boundaries. This is an example of how the ordinarily relied upon guidance of western clinical ethics may not be adequate in complex disaster settings, or at least additional consideration is required to help determine how it can still apply.

3.6 Aid Organisation Statements

In addition to reliance upon professional codes of ethics, humanitarian aid organisations that participate in disaster response often have expressed ethical guidance through value statements. Among them, the International Committee of the Red Cross (ICRC) offers the Fundamental Principles,

- humanity
- impartiality
- neutrality
- independence
- voluntary service
- unity
- universality

Médecins Sans Frontières and Sphere Project (2011), among others, have similarly broad statements that echo some of the values expressed here. Because they are broad value statements they are relevant across multiple settings, strategies and projects. Their breadth also means they tend to succumb to the criticism that the guidance they offer is mostly only useful at higher levels, whereas in particular practical situations in the field, generalised statements offer only vague assistance. In addition, as with many such statements, while each of the values is important, they can conflict when it comes to applying them, and no hierarchy has been established to determine which value will override the others when two or more conflict. For example, responding to a situation of oppression and injustice might override another praiseworthy value such as neutrality, and health practitioners may be ill-prepared to manage the ensuing conflict.

Attempts have been made to clarify the values statements and offer additional guidance to health professionals on how to apply them (Zielinski 1994; Sheather and Shah 2011). This will continue to be necessary to promote understanding of the ethical values and expectations of humanitarian health care organisations. Continual dialogue will be crucial to help understand how ethical requirements ought to be applied, and how best to support ethical responses in disaster settings. The best foundations for this guidance will come from the experiences of field professionals and members of the communities who experience disaster first-hand and can identify best ethical orientations and practices.

3.7 Guidance for Disaster Ethics

In the following sections we propose some concepts and resources from ethical theory and applied ethics that may offer helpful illumination and support for ethical health care practice in disaster settings. This is by no means an exhaustive list, but they are resources that have proven useful during consultations with humanitarian health care practitioners. Among them are questions to help identify an ethical issue when it emerges, concepts borrowed from other fields of applied ethics and other concepts drawn from ethical theory.

3.7.1 Recognising an Ethical Issue

It is reasonable to speculate that there is little time to reflect and acknowledge the presence of ethical challenges during disaster response, or that ethical challenges ought simply to be accepted as inevitable. Some suggest that there are fewer ethical issues in the acute phase because the priority is clearly streamlined toward saving the most lives (Hunt 2009). There may not be time to *recognise* the presence of an ethical issue in the extreme contexts of disaster. However, it is clear that these issues exist, as the respondents echo authors who have described them in their work (Orbinski 2008; Merin et al. 2010). Because of the salience of ethical considerations in providing sound, respectful care in disasters, as in any settings, it is worthwhile considering how to identify ethical challenges when they arise.

For the purposes of the study, we identified ethical challenges as situations when the ethically preferred response is unclear, or clear but could not be enacted. They include situations 'in which each possible course of action breaches some otherwise binding moral principle' (Blackburn 1994, p. 250) or where the respondent perceived that the 'right thing to do' was also wrong in some important way (Schwartz et al. 2010).

An additional question that could trigger identification of an ethical issue is to ask, Who will be harmed by a decision and who stands to benefit? In disaster settings social disparities and injustices will be pronounced or newly emerge. In such cases it may not always be evident who stands to be harmed by a decision, especially when choices need to be made urgently, with little time to consider long-term outcomes. Taking the time to become conscious of who will benefit from a decision and what will be the resulting harms is potentially illuminating and can help prevent problems before they arise.[2]

The case discussed above yields some important considerations for health care professionals and the aid agencies they travel with. Thus our findings indicate that four additional interconnected questions ought to be addressed before a mission begins:

1. What are the needs of the people in the disaster setting?
2. What are my intentions for going?
3. What is the aim of the mission for the aid agency?
4. Do the responses to (1), (2) and (3) harmonise?

The first of these questions is critical and will be considered in more detail below. The second and third questions can help the professionals clarify and reflect upon the goals, expectations and limitations of the kind of care that can be provided during a mission. If health practitioners are clear about the mission and its limits they will be able to determine in advance whether their intentions coincide with those of the aid agency. If there is a disparity between their respective intentions, then an ethical dilemma is a real likelihood in the field. Thus, surgeon may see it as their duty to treat a patient's hernia when other pressing disaster-related surgical cases are not present, while the aid organisation may be committed to preserving its limited resources for patients who were injured in the disaster. The health professionals will then need to consider whether and to what extent they are prepared to accept the mission of the aid agency and permit it to become their priority. Of course, in the end, if neither the intentions of the health professionals nor the aims of the mission are relevant to the needs of the disaster victims, then an additional ethical challenge will be easily identifiable.

Once an ethical challenge is identified, there is also the matter of identifying the right means with which to report, examine or debate the matter.

3.7.2 Evidence Base and A Lesson from Research Ethics

An ethically relevant feature of disaster settings is that they are rapidly shifting and thus laden with uncertainty. In particular for health care practice, great gaps tend to exist in knowledge of how best to treat the injuries that occur during natural disasters.

[2] We also suggest the following useful questions proposed by ethics scholars at Santa Clara University (Markkula Center for Applied Ethics 2009):

- Could this decision or situation be damaging to someone or to some group?
- Does this decision involve a choice between a good and bad alternative, or perhaps between two "goods" or between two "bads"?
- Is this issue about more than what is legal or what is most efficient? If so, how?

Only a fledgling evidence base exists for disaster medicine because of the many barriers to conducting robust research in these settings. Treatment can consist of n-of-1 experimentation or small hopeful trials of interventions devised for the constraints and difficulties that emerge from a given disaster. Recently, ethical concerns have begun to emerge about this kind of evidence-generating approach to care in disaster situations. These include questions about the ability of patient participants to give informed consent while dealing with the trauma and loss resulting from the disaster; or how to find adequately constituted research ethics review bodies in the aftermath of devastating natural phenomena. These are significant issues that are addressed elsewhere (O'Mathúna 2010) so we will not go over them here. Instead we wish to draw upon a concept from research ethics that could provide useful direction for ethics in humanitarian health care practice as well.

In the Council for International Organizations of Medical Sciences (CIOMS) statement on international research ethics, researchers who work with vulnerable populations are called upon to be *responsive* to local needs. The CIOMS statement describes particular details of how this can be carried out, not least of which is through consultation with the local community to help determine its perceived needs and priorities (CIOMS 2009, guideline 10).

A similar conception of *responsiveness* is crucial for the provision of care in disaster settings, where *merely* responding in the sense of 'just showing up with the desire to help' may be less fruitful than more meaningful kinds of responsiveness. Naturally, context will be relevant because responsiveness will be different in the immediate relief phase as opposed to the following weeks, so priorities may be reconsidered once the acutely injured have been treated. This indicates that an ethical requirement for humanitarian health care practice should be responsiveness in the following ways: it ought to involve responsible preparedness in the form both of needs assessments *and* consultation; in other words, a willingness to find out from the community representatives of the disaster what the community's priority needs are, as opposed to merely making assumptions about their needs. Then, the organisation and practitioners can offer relevant interventions, which respond to the perceived needs of the population and patients in question. This does not mean foregoing an independent assessment of the situation, but being sure that more local information is used in decision-making about the best way to provide and prioritise resources. In isolation a unilateral needs-assessment is useful but incomplete. This means that aid organisations and health practitioners must make the effort to understand what is required of them to support local leadership in making fair prioritisation decisions. Otherwise, merely showing up can be wasteful and even dangerous.

Responsiveness can help avoid creating additional problems that an already overburdened system will be left to solve, such as safely disposing of expired or irrelevant medications sent by well-meaning donors who do not take the time to be sure their donation is relevant. Meaningful responsiveness, which combines responsiveness to community-identified needs with evidence-based needs-assessment, is a useful guiding concept because it appeals to aid organisations and health care practitioners to offer assistance that is carefully measured to be of use to the community in need, for example that they have the right mix of skills and equipment to address local needs. It cannot alleviate all problems however, such as situations where the perceived need is in conflict with what the health care professionals say is the evidence-based need. For example, in one case, the humanitarian health care providers prioritised the children in an under-5 infant mortality campaign, but local community members questioned this plan as they thought the elders should be prioritised. In this case further ethical dilemmas would need to be addressed.

3.7.3 Ideal and Non-ideal Approaches to Ethical Challenges

A theoretical concept that may be helpfully employed in disaster bioethics is the distinction between *ideal* and *non-ideal* moral theory. Applied health care ethics is highly influenced by ideal theory that attempts to offer practical guidance, based on values and principles, to inform ethical action. As Lisa Tessman puts it, idealised moral theorists posit that, 'Moral goodness is always possible; one is never forced to leave a moral requirement (that is still in force) unfulfilled' (2010, p. 801). Tessman is critical of this optimistic perspective because she says it fails to acknowledge the imperfections that impact real world actions, such as oppression and injustice. Ideal theory is focused on generating normative statements that assert a best choice, all things being equal, but is ill-equipped to provide guidance on how to go from real life imperfect situations to ideal ones. In contrast, non-ideal ethics begins with a description of the circumstances of an event, which includes an account of complicating factors such as oppression and past injustices. Non-ideal theory starts from 'what is the case' and then either proposes guidance for improvement, or acknowledges that the dilemma is irresolvable under current oppressive conditions.

> ... there are times when a normative theory cannot point triumphantly at anything good or right. I think that truly recognizing the fact of oppression entails acknowledging the associated failures of morality. (Tessman 2010, p. 798)

In situations such as disaster and complex humanitarian emergencies, non-ideal theory can offer two important elements. First, it begins with descriptive detail of a given situation, which takes into account the injustices of the context, past and present. Second, non-ideal theory acknowledges the irresolvability of some ethical dilemmas because of the injustices present and the inescapable need to choose between, and therefore necessarily violate, important guiding values and ethical principles. The first point is arguably more relevant in some contexts than in others. It is more applicable when natural disasters coincide with political oppression or armed conflict. Nevertheless non-ideal moral theory would identify as relevant even comparatively mild or limited social oppression, so few cases would be entirely free from oppression.

The second feature of non-ideal theory, acceptance of irresolvable ethical dilemmas, is likely to be relevant in any disaster because of the nature of the events which by definition involve failure, crisis, loss, hardship and destruction. The respondents in our study related multiple stories of circumstances where no ideal answer could be given to the ethical challenge and they felt any response would in some way violate another significant moral value or duty. This could account for the feelings of powerlessness the respondents described as they went on missions feeling empowered to help, worked enormously hard, and still felt they had not done enough.

In the case described above, the actors were forced to choose between competing duties: the duty to comply with agency policies and protocols in order to respect country mandates and donor wishes and the clinicians' duty of care toward this person whom they perceived as a 'patient' and felt an obligation to assist. None of these are trivial, as the former is the means by which aid agencies can continue their work in agreement with local governments and funders, while the latter is their reason for being there to begin with. Again, this is no trivial obligation as clinicians owe a duty of care to their patients as stated in their professional codes of ethics (e.g. WMA), but also because this man's ability to work as a farmer was the only means he had to provide food for his family. A simple list of obligations would offer no useful guidance in this case unless it had a defined hierarchy to instantiate which was the most important duty to respect. A relevant morally binding principle will be breached either way, so non-ideal theory helps acknowledge the inevitable moral failure of these sorts of situations, or what Alex de Waal (2010) called the 'inescapable cruelties' of humanitarian aid. Perhaps this is cold-comfort, but an important acknowledgment nonetheless, as it reflects the realities reported by aid workers, and validates their sense of powerlessness to provide care for all who need it.

Non-ideal theory is useful, but contains the potential flaw that it may discourage actors from even attempting to resolve an ethical dilemma that they may wrongly perceive as hopeless. It should not be an excuse for inaction, but a catalyst for recognising when a different approach is required, one that attempts to rectify injustice but does not perceive the persistence of moral imperfection as a failure. An alternate approach to the case, for example, might be to address when it is that disaster relief work transforms into other categories of humanitarian aid such as reconstruction or development. If the aid agency in this case could have resolved that the crisis had shifted from immediate disaster to rebuilding, it may have been possible to reorder their priorities as well. Nine weeks after the initial event, it was possible that medical needs directly caused by the event would have already been addressed. Whereas the destruction of the health care system was an on-going crisis, so non-disaster related medical needs could have become the new guiding priority for the mission. This would have involved renegotiation of their presence and the use of donor funds, as well as an additional effort to organise and plan an exit strategy to ensure the mission rebuilt and did not become a substitute for the naturalised health care system.

3.8 An Ethics Analysis Tool to Support Decision-making

It can be helpful for health care practitioners working in disaster settings to be able to draw upon tools and frameworks for addressing ethical challenges they encounter in the field. Elsewhere, we have presented a detailed ethics analysis tool to support

Table 3.1 Humanitarian Health Ethics Analysis Tool

hhe humanitarian healthcare ethics
reflecting on ethical practice

Humanitarian Ethics Analysis Tool

1. **Identify/clarify ethical Issue:**
   What is at stake and for whom?
2. **Gather Information:**
   What do we need to know to assess the issue?
3. **Review Ethical Issue:**
   Does information gathered lead us to reformulate the issue?
4. **Explore ethics resources:**
   What can help us make a decision?
5. **Evaluate and select the best option:**
   What options are possible and which is the "best" under the circumstances?
6. **Follow up:** What can we learn from this situation, what supports are needed?

htp://www.humanitarianhealthethics.net/

hhe humanitarian healthcare ethics
reflecting on ethical practice

Humanitarian Ethics Analysis Tool	
1.	Is this truly an ethical issue? What is at stake & for whom? How is the issue perceived from different perspectives? When must a decision be made? Who is responsible for making it? What has been done so far?
2.	What information is needed to deliberate well about this issue and enable us to make a well-considered decision? What constraints to information gathering exist? Consider: a) Participation, perspectives and power b) Community, project and policies c) Resources, clinical features & obstacles
3.	Does the process so far reveal new aspects of the ethical issue or suggest the need to reformulate or redefine the issue? Have our biases/interests affected how we see the issue?
4.	What can assist us to evaluate the ethical aspects of this issue? What values and norms ought to inform our decision making? Consider: Codes of ethics (NGO, interagency, professional bodies); local & international law; statements of values/principles; agency policies
5.	What options are possible in this situation and what ethical values support each option? What consequences might result from each option? Can consequences, values and obligations be reconciled?
6.	What can we learn from this situation? What support do those involved need?

http://www.humanitarianhealthethics.net/

decision-making in humanitarian health care practice that draws upon existing models used in other domains of health care (Hunt 2011). The tool offers a set of questions to keep in mind when responding to an ethical challenge. It derives from ethical theory more broadly, but is built upon the cases and experiences of humanitarian health care providers in emergency response and other realms of humanitarian aid. An updated and abbreviated version of the Humanitarian Health Ethics Analysis Tool (HHEAT) is presented in Table 3.1 and an accompanying handbook is in development. The elements of the tool are meant to guide discussion or reflection in a manner which is sensitive to the ethically relevant details in the case.[3]

Even in urgent response situations these kinds of questions can be a resource for practitioners, unit managers and policy makers. The questions can be applied in the field or prior to departure, and could be included in broader decision-making. In addition, we have found the tool useful when applied to cases in pre-departure training. The questions may also be helpful upon return from the field. They can provide a mechanism for discussion and reflection upon difficult issues that arose so that clinicians can learn from experiences and communicate what they have learned.

---

[3] More information on the tool can be found at: www.humanitarianhealthethics.net. We would like to acknowledge Veronique Fraser for the work she has put into validating and clarifying this tool.

3.9 Case 2: After the Earthquake

Eight weeks after the earthquake in Haiti, humanitarian health care practitioners were working at a field hospital about two hours outside of the capital Port-au-Prince. One late afternoon, an acutely sick baby was brought in with respiratory distress. The field hospital had neither the personnel nor the equipment to actively care for this condition. The child needed to be transferred to another facility in Port au Prince. A curfew of 6 pm was in place for the team and it was now about 3:30 pm. The drive would take about two or two-and-a-half hours if the roads were clear and there was not too much traffic, so the people who accompanied the baby would not be able to return until the next day. The stretch of road to Port au Prince was also a dangerous kidnapping area.

Because of the time of day, using a vehicle to transport the baby meant leaving the team with only one vehicle overnight. This was against unit protocol because one vehicle was not enough to evacuate the team if that was needed due to an aftershock or for security reasons. The doctor asked the unit manager if they could use the vehicle to transport the baby anyway.

In this case, once again, questions emerge about the loyalties, duties and expectations of humanitarian health care practice. Clinical knowledge of what could be done with resources available in the health providers' home context was thwarted by the absence of the resources in the field hospital. If the baby could be transferred the doctor would have been able to fulfil what was perceived to be duty of care to the patient. However, the responsibility of the unit manager was directed toward the security of the team. Though multiple other complexities surrounded the event, at the heart of the case was a conflict of loyalties and trade-offs that needed to be made. The security of the team coupled with uncertainties about the safety of travel, the possibility the doctor might be kidnapped or the baby would not survive the trip raised the stakes, and there was no guarantee the hospital in the city would have a functioning ventilator available for this child anyway. On the other hand, the doctor saw a clear path toward helping the baby survive and knew there was no other option than to look for assistance in the city.

Two valuable goals were presented, with no way to assure both would be achieved other than taking a chance by transporting the baby and hope the team would not need to evacuate during the hours the doctor was gone. In this case an assured harm—the death of the child—was measured against the risk that many staff could be harmed if a sudden evacuation was required overnight before the doctor could return with the vehicle. What if the gamble did not pay off?

3.10 Making and Maintaining Moral Space for Ethical Debate

Respondents in the study all described at least three situations of this sort, where ethical challenges had emerged in their work, and some talked about ethical experience more broadly. They recounted stories that belied a sense of responsibility to act to improve situations, in particular when they believed patient care was compromised by ethical challenges. They also talked about the courage needed to respond.

> In the name of ethics, you can challenge medical policies. You can challenge, which is great, but, I mean, it takes a lot of courage.

Moral courage accounts for how and whether individuals respond in ethical challenges (Sekerka and Bagozzin 2007), but the moral courage of individuals cannot be enough because it implies that responsibility falls to single actors to intervene in ethical conflict. Individuals will be responsible for responding, but they should not bear this responsibility alone. There needs to be an accepted culture within aid contexts and organisations, supported by formal structures, for addressing ethical challenges either right away or in critical incident analyses. A culture of ethical reflection will permit more natural deliberation, can reduce conflict and, most importantly, can improve responses to ethical disputes that may put patients, practitioners and missions at risk.

> When I worked with [aid agency] suddenly the support was there. I was able to sit down around a table and have pizza with people that have worked in camps in Goma or during the siege in Sierra Leone. Just to listen to their stories suddenly I felt like I was in the community that I felt very comfortable with sharing these things. And that now we're a team . . . even though I was away from the base by hundreds of miles, I felt quite close and that I knew I didn't have to make decisions alone. And that whatever we, whatever the issue was we could come together to make the best decision together.

Within teams and organisations, practical opportunities can be established to facilitate space for ethics in humanitarian health care practice. Local teams can use regular time in meetings and mentoring to encourage discussion that will help share the weight of ethical issues and management of challenges as they arise. Similar resources should be employed in broader organisational practices, permitting ethical reflection to move from the background to regular reflective application of values in practice.

In pre-departure training, team members can be prepared to face ethical challenges by giving them time to discuss cases and through the discussions identify ways in which intentions, duties and expectations can conflict to create ethical tensions. The discussion may not be able to cover all types of problems they encounter, but it does create an opportunity to see how discussions can unfold and how models and ethically oriented considerations can improve responses.

The values statements of organisations like ICRC, MSF and Sphere are useful resources for understanding what is anticipated and expected of those participating in field missions. The theoretical concepts we have described here are also meant to help all stakeholders anticipate, respond and adjust to the non-ideal realities of humanitarian care in disaster settings. We hope that these, together with application of the HHEAT tool, offer some useful foundations for education and reflection on ethical challenges arising in humanitarian healthcare. More work should be done to develop further resources and a common framework for applied ethics in this context.

3.11 Conclusion

We have attempted to demonstrate the value of ethics training for health care practitioners involved in disaster response. Respondents in our study acknowledged this as a means of priming them to manage ethical challenges in the field, or ideally avoid them altogether. As one respondent put it, ethics education,

> . . . may not have helped me in the senses that I knew what was right and what was wrong but it helped me in the sense that I knew what to do for support. That I knew that I didn't have to make a decision by myself right now, that I had a whole network of support that I could call upon and that I should call upon in fact and give regular updates too. Because this is a team mission I'm not by myself.

The stories of ethical challenges collected in our study provide the early stages of an empirical base for understanding what ethical conflicts humanitarian health care practitioners encountered in the field. The resources for supporting ethical humanitarian health care are potentially numerous. Those we have described here have three origins: first from formal qualitative collection and analysis of stories of ethical challenges encountered by health professionals in the field; second, from their recommendations for the kinds of resources they either usefully employed or anticipated being helpful (Hunt et al. 2012); and third, from existing and emerging concepts in ethical theory and scholarship. Further work needs to be done to create a full set of resources to help prepare and support ethical humanitarian health care practice. Most significantly, these resources will remain incomplete until the perspectives of local health professionals, patients and communities are added (Sumathipala et al. 2010). Ideally, collaboration between all the players and stakeholders will be brought together to inform this emerging stream of applied ethics.

References

Blackburn, S. 1994. *The Oxford dictionary of philosophy*. Oxford: Oxford University Press.

CIOMS. 2009. International ethical guidelines for epidemiological studies Council for International Organizations of Medical Sciences.

Costello, Amy. 2012. Medical volunteers learn from mistakes made in Haiti. Public Radio International, October 12. http://www.pri.org/stories/health/global-health/medical-volunteers-learn-from-mistakes-made-in-rush-to-haiti-11761.html. Accessed 24 June 2013.

De Waal, Alex. 2010. The humanitarians' tragedy: Escapable and inescapable cruelties. *Disasters* 34 (Suppl 2): S130–S137.

DuVal, Gordon, Leah Sartorius, Brian Clarridge, Gary Gensler, and Marion Danis. 2001. What triggers requests for ethics consultations? *Journal of Medical Ethics* 27 (Suppl 1): i24–i29.

Etienne, M., C. Powell, and D. Amundson. 2010. Healthcare ethics: The experience after the Haitian earthquake. *American Journal of Disaster Medicine* 5 (3): 141–147.

Fox, Ellen, Sarah Myers, and Robert A. Pearlman. 2007. Ethics consultation in United States hospitals: A national survey. *American Journal of Bioethics* 7 (2): 13–25.

Hunt, Matthew R. 2009. Resources and constraints for addressing ethical issues in medical humanitarian work: Experiences of expatriate healthcare professionals. *American Journal of Disaster Medicine* 4 (5): 261–271.

Hunt, Matthew R. 2011. Establishing moral bearings: Ethics and expatriate health care professionals in humanitarian work. *Disasters* 35 (3): 606–622.

Hunt, M. R., L. Schwartz, and L. Elit. 2012. Ethics support and training for health professionals in international aid work. *Public Health Ethics* 5 (1): 91–99.

Markkula Center for Applied Ethics. 2009. A framework for thinking ethically. http://www.scu.edu/ethics/practicing/decision/framework.html. Accessed 15 July 2011.

Merin, Ofer, Nachman Ash, Gad Levy, Mitchell J. Schwaber, and Yitshak Kreiss. 2010. The Israeli field hospital in Haiti—Ethical dilemmas in early disaster response. *New England Journal of Medicine* 362 (11): e38.

Médecins Sans Frontières. 2013. MSF Charter. http://www.msf.ca/about-msf/msf-charter/. Accessed 1 May 2013.

O'Mathúna, Dónal P. 2010. Conducting research in the aftermath of disasters: Ethical considerations. *Journal of Evidence Based Medicine* 3:65–75.

Orbinski, James. 2008. *An imperfect offering: Humanitarian action in the twenty-first century*. Toronto: Doubleday Canada.

Redwood-Campbell, L. J., and L. Riddez. 2006. Post-tsunami medical care: Health problems encountered in the International Committee of the Red Cross hospital in Banda Aceh, Indonesia. *Prehospital & Disaster Medicine* 21 (1): s1–s7.

Schwartz, Lisa, Christina Sinding, Matthew Hunt, Laurie Elit, Lynda Redwood-Campbell, Naomi Adelson, Lori Luther, Jennifer Ranford, and Sonya de Laat. 2010. Ethics in humanitarian aid work: Learning from the narratives of humanitarian health workers. *American Journal of Bioethics: Primary Research* 1 (3): 45–54.

Schwartz, Lisa, Matthew R. Hunt, Chris Sinding, Laurie Elit, Lynda Redwoord-Campbell, Naomi Adelson, and Sonya de Laat. 2012. Models for humanitarian health care ethics. *Public Health Ethics* 5 (1): 81–90.

Sekerka, Leslie E., and Richard P. Bagozzin. 2007. Moral courage in the workplace: moving to and from the desire and decision to act. *Business Ethics: A European Review* 16 (2): 132–149.

Sheather, Julian, and Tejshri Shah. 2011. Ethical dilemmas in medical humanitarian practice: cases for reflection from Médecins Sans Frontières. *Journal of Medical Ethics* 37:162–165.

Sinding, Christina, Lisa Schwartz, Matthew Hunt, Linda Redwood-Campbell, Laurie Elit, and Jennifer Ranford. 2010. 'Playing God because you have to': Health professionals' narratives of rationing care in humanitarian and development work. *Public Health Ethics* 3 (2): 147–156.

Sontag, Deborah. 2010. Doctors haunted by Haitians they couldn't help. New York Times, February 12. http://www.nytimes.com/2010/02/13/world/americas/13doctors.html. Accessed 24 June 2013.

Sphere, Project. 2011. Humanitarian Charter and Minimum Standards in Humanitarian Response. United Kingdom: Practical Action Publishing Company. http://www.sphereproject.org/handbook/. Accessed 1 May 2013.

Sumathipala, Athula, Amir Jafarey, Leonardo D. de Castro, Aasim Ahmad, Darryl Marcer, Sandya Srinivasan, Nandini Kumar, Sisira Siribaddana, Sleman Sutaryo, Anant Bhan, Dananjaya Waidyaratne, Sriyakanthi Beneragama, Chandrani Jayasekera, Sarath Edirisingha, and Chesmal Siriwardhana. 2010. Ethical issues in post-disaster clinical interventions and research: A developing world perspective. Key findings from a drafting and consensus generation meeting of the Working Group on Disaster Research and Ethics (WGDRE) 2007. *Asian Bioethics Review* 2 (2): 124–142.

Tessman, Lisa. 2010. Idealizing Morality. *Hypatia* 25 (4): 797–824.

World Medical Association. 2006. WMA statement on medical ethics in the event of disasters. World Medical Association.

Zielinski, Henryk. 1994. Health and humanitarian concerns: Principles and ethics. Springer.

Chapter 4
Triage in Disaster Medicine: Ethical Strategies in Various Scenarios

Y. Michael Barilan, Margherita Brusa and Pinchas Halperin

Disaster scenarios are divided into three prototypes—disasters visiting well-ordered societies, disruptive disasters that wreak havoc on the infrastructure of society, and "double disasters" that ravage poor societies whose infrastructure had already been substantially deficient. Three prototypical schemes of triage are described—the "utilitarian", the "clinical" and a "hybrid" of the two. It is argued that all three are ethically reasonable, although some seem to be more applicable to certain disaster scenarios.

4.1 Introduction

A medical team arrives in a disaster stricken area. It is working as hard as it can, saving lives, reducing disability and alleviating suffering. The physical efforts are taxing, the psychological stress is pressing, and the moral distress is excruciating. So, why do dedicated caregivers, who save lives and help victims, suffer morally at all? Conversations with rescue teams bring forth the agony of triage. Relief workers and healthcare professionals are troubled by "no treatment" decisions and are haunted by flashbacks of rejected victims. The selection of patients for treatment—either in terms of priority (who is first) or principle (who will be treated at all)—is known as triage. This use of the word was initiated by the Surgeon General of Napoleon's Imperial Guard in order to systematise medical care in the battlefield (Burris et al. 2004; Winslow 1982).

Although triage is principally a question of allocation of vital resources, the special circumstances of disaster medicine render triage in disaster care a special sub-set of

Y. M. Barilan (✉)
Department of Medical Education, Sackler School of Medicine,
Tel Aviv University, Tel Aviv, Israel
e-mail: ymbarilan@gmail.com

M. Brusa
Department of Pediatrics, University of Padua, Padua, Italy

P. Halperin
Tel Aviv Medical Center, Tel Aviv, Israel

D. P. O'Mathúna et al. (eds.), *Disaster Bioethics: Normative Issues When Nothing is Normal,* Public Health Ethics Analysis 2, DOI 10.1007/978-94-007-3864-5_4,

moral, clinical and psychological problems. We focus on the ethics of clinical triage performed by medical teams in arenas of humanitarian disaster. We will argue that the circumstances of disaster bear directly in the ethics of triage and that different triage strategies fit different disaster settings.

First, we will divide disasters into three prototypical scenarios. Second, on the basis of actual practice and the literature we will explicate three prototypical schemes of triage—the "utilitarian", the "clinical" and a "hybrid" version. We examine the suitability of the schemes to the prototypical scenarios and will argue that the "hybrid" version is usually most reasonable clinically, morally and psychologically. Prior to the conclusion we will present in detail how the "hybrid" scheme works.

This chapter deals with natural disasters such as earthquakes, tsunamis and volcanic eruptions as well as non-natural disasters such as the September 11th attacks in the US. Common to these situations is the absence of complicating factors such as the conditions in a battlefield. In the "simple" disasters under discussion here, the factors in play are the victims, the caring teams, the available resources, and the background material and social conditions. Triage in war and other armed conflicts may raise unique ethical questions (Gross 2006). Triage during epidemics often involves two fundamental conflicts of loyalty— the first conflict arises because the victims are both patients and sources of contagion; the second arises from healthcare professionals' duty to care for victims but also the value of protecting one's self and family. As others have addressed the ethics of care during biological warfare and pandemics (Iserson and Pesik 2003; Kass et al. 2008) we will not consider these here. Neither will we explore the limits of medical altruism, for example, when, if at all, medical personnel may fly away to safer places, leaving the needy behind (Iserson 2008).

4.2 Mapping out Disasters

4.2.1 Well Circumscribed Disasters

A well circumscribed disaster is one which occurs within a society that otherwise functions well in terms of material and political culture. Although Rawls had political structure and not material culture in mind, these circumstances fit roughly his notion of "well-ordered society" (Rawls 1971, p. 397). A paradigmatic example would be the attack on the Twin Towers on September 11, 2001. The victims had not suffered from neglect or extreme poverty before the attack, and the shortage in basic care was perceived as technical and temporary. In well circumscribed disasters, provision of optimum care is mainly a race against time. A well intentioned passer-by may tend to a victim or a group of victims; but healthcare professionals operate within their roles as members of professional teams entrusted by the public. They are morally committed to all victims alike (as well as to potential victims and the public at large). The more opportunities and capabilities, the broader and deeper is the moral responsibility to save and to medically help as many people as possible. This is true of any person, but the professional can do more and the professional is also bounded by the internal morality of the profession; she may have to obey orders to continue driving to a specific site, passing by needy people on the way.

In well circumscribed disasters "conventional triage" may be appropriate. As Gross explains, 'During conventional triage, medical supplies are ample so that supplies are properly managed, medical personnel can successfully treat all of the wounded.... This translates into first treating those whose injuries are most severe' (Gross 2006, p. 145). Since policies of "conventional triage" are rife and relatively noncontroversial, this paper analyses "mass causality triage", when it is evident that a substantial number of victims cannot be treated and saved, no matter what strategy of triage and organisation of care is deployed ("non-Pareto optimal contexts").

A variant of well circumscribed disasters occurs when a well-ordered society is lacking one or a few essential components of therapy, for example, vaccinations, dialysis machines or respirators. The healthcare system is otherwise intact and is capable of offering other aspects of care (at least at the basic level) to all. The recent literature on resource allocation in pandemics addresses this kind of problem.

4.2.2 *Disruptive Disasters*

A second kind of disaster disrupts the fabric of social life and its material infrastructure. Such disruptions include massive blockage of roads, blackout of electricity and communication services, loss of water supply and waste treatment facilities, as well as loss of personal safety due to looting and general disorder. Harsh weather conditions may exacerbate these damages significantly. In disruptive disasters, effective clinical care (even if somehow delayed) depends on immediate shunting of resources for the sake of repairing infrastructure and public order. Clinicians are expected (or ordered) to accept compromise in clinical care and in ethics because society as a whole is mobilised for the sake of the victims and for the sake of prevention of a secondary disaster of larger magnitude than the original one. It is also noteworthy that reinstatement of public health and order are necessary for the provision of clinical care.

In less extreme cases, the disruption is partial, pushing the healthcare system to downgrade significantly its standards of care due to the combination of physical damage and increased patient load.

4.2.3 *Double Disasters*

A third paradigmatic disaster occurs when an already impoverished and unstable society sustains a sharp increase in destruction, death and injury. Although the very notion of disaster conveys an abrupt and destructive disruption of ordinary life, double disasters occur when the disrupted routine is already chaotic, perilous and full of misery. Owing to poor infrastructure, the destructive impact of double disasters is immense. Indeed, poor infrastructure and corrupt governments render the population even more susceptible to calamity. In double disasters, response almost always depends on foreign humanitarian aid and the gap between its capacity to help and the burden of injury is huge.

Although all large scale disasters threaten to dehumanise the afflicted societies (Sorokin 1942), the typically exotic, distant and disorderly nature of double disaster locations are particularly susceptible to inadvertent but unacceptable practices that dehumanise the victims. Well intentioned healthcare professionals should be alert to the inadvertent impacts of their actions on the human face of society (International Federation of Red Cross 1995). This entails concern about protection of privacy against prurient photography and the setting of clear boundaries between the sphere of the clinic and the media.

4.3 An Outline for Schemes of Triage in Disaster Medicine

4.3.1 Utilitarian Schemes for Mass Casualty Triage

Within the utilitarian scheme, every triage decision is made solely following consideration of maximising medical benefit overall. With disasters, there is a strong utilitarian case in favour of granting priority to reduction of suffering and loss over the promotion of health and happiness ("the asymmetric thesis"; see Mayerfeld 1999).

In the face of death and agony, there is a strong case for defining "medical goals" as comprised of three endpoints: (1) saving life, not merely deferring death by days or even weeks; (2) reduction of suffering; and (3) reduction of long term morbidity and disability. A utilitarian scheme would grant higher priority to saving life that is not doomed to extreme suffering and then to reduction of suffering and long term disability. But these medical goals are often incommensurate with each other. Hence, within the utilitarian paradigm there are different, even competing methods for defining utility. One may count the number of lives saved regardless of future life expectancy. In this manner, saving an eighty year old person counts as much as saving a baby. It is also possible to count life-years earned, factoring in the gain in longevity or even the gain in quality-adjusted life years (QALYs). Alternatively, one may argue that the scarce good to be distributed is not lives or life-years saved, but the chance to recover or to escape agony. In this light, every non-trivially and non-fatally injured person has an equal claim to care. When resources are rationed, we should allocate portions to every segment of society, covering different stages of the life cycle (Emanuel and Wertheimer 2006)). In the same vein, one may argue for some preferential regard for people with special needs, who would otherwise die and suffer disproportionally to their prevalence in society (without basic help, they will remain under the rubble, blind, deaf, disabled, psychotic or handicapped).

The incorporation of such considerations will thicken the prevailing utilitarian guidelines that address the number of lives saved in the short run. Additionally, this will result in more than one reasonable utilitarian scheme (White et al. 2009). Indeed, different societies have different historical heritages and different approaches to "tragic choices" (Calabresi and Bobbit 1978). Utilitarian medicine in general depends on society and culture in order to formulate the goods to be promoted—what constitutes "well-being" and "medical benefit" for the given people in a given context. Ultimately, even within a utilitarian framework, public deliberation becomes the most reasonable means to provide legitimacy to the triage strategy that will be adopted (Fleck 2009).

The common denominator of all utilitarian schemes is the commitment to fairly maximise a pre-defined medical good among all relevant persons (i.e. victims within reach). With the exception of the taboo on sacrificing one person for the sake of others, this commitment overrides all other moral considerations, especially those related to the individual doctor-patient relationship, such as fiduciary commitments.[1] Within the utilitarian scheme, the loyalty of the healthcare professionals is owed solely to the fair promotion of medical good among all reachable victims. According to the utilitarian scheme, in disaster medicine, despite the personal doctor/nurse-patient relationship, the true patient of care is all medically treatable victims. Put in other words, the utilitarian scheme of triage in disaster medicine combines public health with clinical care.

The utilitarian scheme requires the transfer of resources from low-prognosis patients to high-prognosis patients. In ordinary situations, it is usually viewed as immoral to disconnect a patient from a respirator or discontinue a therapeutic program in order to make the treatment available for a more promising patient. Many regard this as a breach of loyalty to the first patient. It may be argued that in disaster medicine, loyalty to individual patients in terms of resource allocation is weaker than in ordinary medicine. Whereas in ordinary circumstances the free and personal relationship between doctor and patient is the basis of clinical ethics, in disaster medicine the overall ethics of disaster care predicates the interpersonal relationship between individual caregivers and their patients. The personal duties of doctors to patients are contingent upon the doctors' humanitarian commitment to the community of victims as a whole. Therefore, in disaster medicine fair and judicious shift of resources from one patient to another does not constitute patient abandonment, even if the outcome is the death of the first patient.

There could be a utilitarian argument defending triage schemes that grants preference to the care of a class of persons fulfilling socially important roles (police, fire-fighters, healthcare professionals, etc.). Some military triage schemes for conditions of active combat grant the highest priority to the care of injured soldiers who may return to fight (so called "reverse triage"; see Gross 2006).

The utilitarian scheme suffers from three chief difficulties. First, due to the extreme and unpredictable circumstances of disaster, not only treatment resources are lacking, but also instruments of monitoring, follow-up and quality control. Caregivers will

[1] We do not explore here the philosophical question of whether utilitarianism endorses the deliberate sacrifice of the few for the sake of saving the many (e.g. the question of "survival lottery"). Since no healthcare system in the world practices sacrificial care, we take this de-facto taboo as a given.

count the patients seen and procedures done (if they have enough writing material), being ignorant of the real numbers ultimately helped. The shorter the period of care, the more efficient it might seem; but in the absence of follow-up and evidence-based resources, the utilitarian scheme is at risk of being self-defeating. Since doctors and nurses are unlikely either to be trained in or familiar with shifting resources from one patient to another, such actions may create an impression of efficiency, while in actuality, they prevent successful care reaching everybody. Those rejected during triage will be left uncared for; those whose care is compromised by utilitarian modifications of the standards of good care, will not be able to benefit either. Since utilitarian justifications depend wholly on objective and measurable outcomes, this is a very serious drawback.

Second, the three chief utilitarian medical goods (i.e. life, reduction of morbidity and disability, and alleviation of suffering) are not readily commensurable. It is not clear whether purely utilitarian considerations can determine whether to save many lives, but with reduced functionality or quality of life (for example, by means of amputations) or to save fewer lives, with improved functionality (e.g. contusion of the lung, rhabdomyolysis). In the absence of utilitarian reasons to choose one scheme of action rather than another, policy makers are pushed beyond utilitarian considerations (Barilan 2004). If we are doubtful about the ability of the utilitarian scheme to save more lives (or promote other utilitarian goals) relative to other schemes, and if we cannot tell which utilitarian scheme is the most appropriate morally, the moral authority of utilitarianism shrinks considerably.

Third, if we have strict utilitarianism in mind, every action should promote health. Put in other words, every course of action that brings forth an outcome that contains higher rates of mortality, morbidity and suffering relative to the alternatives is immoral. Yet, strict utilitarianism threatens to destabilise known practices of care. For example, from a utilitarian perspective it might make sense to distribute morphine to those rejected by triage so as to ameliorate their lingering agony and death, at the expense of patients selected for life-saving care. It may be proposed that more suffering will be averted by efficient pain control for the many that are doomed to die than by offering it to the few whose lives and health are being restored by means of surgery and medical care. We conjecture that such policies of care will be found absurd and psychologically too difficult to bear. Doctors and nurses will not operate on victims without anaesthesia or pain control, the utilitarian benefits to other sufferers notwithstanding. Subjecting every medical policy and decision to the utilitarian test will transform all medical care into a gigantic triage calculation that continuously reconsiders whether each medical station (e.g. operating theatre, recovery, post-surgical care) is occupied by the most promising patients and whether every aspect of care (e.g. every dosage of morphine or antibiotics) is justified. The unrelenting utilitarian pressure to optimise is a well-known problem. When added to the psychological burden of disaster care, it might be overwhelming, even for altruistic doctors who might wish to do everything for the sake human life.

4.3.2 Clinical Schemes of Triage in Mass Casualty Disasters

We will call the second scheme of care "clinical", because it is derived from ordinary clinical ethics, in ways that ignore the extraordinary circumstances of disaster. Within this scheme, healthcare professionals reject only the obviously mild and the undoubtedly hopeless cases. All other patients may be admitted on the basis of available occupancy following fair criteria, such as "first come, first served". Proponents of the clinical scheme refuse to assume utilitarian responsibilities for crowds of victims that are extremely disproportionate to the meagre healthcare resources. They care for whoever comes their way, and as long as they are busy with current patients they do not feel responsible for others, no matter what their needs and prognoses.

However, since the role of triage in the clinical scheme is marginal (it only rejects non-medical cases, very mild injuries and the obviously hopeless victims), caregivers are likely to face needy patients empty handed. They will try to care for a newborn baby despite not having appropriate equipment, and to offer ICU care but no dialysis to crash victims with acute renal failure. The higher the ratio of victims to medical resources, the more clinical schemes are at risk of wavering between the occasional heroic (sophisticated and prolonged fight for the life of one person) and the banal provision of very basics of care (painkillers, antibiotics, wound dressing and fixations). The medical team will not suffer the pain of rejecting needy people, but it will suffer witnessing their most precious resources (e.g. respirators, surgical capacities) being wasted.

One may expect that within the clinical scheme, triage is easiest and simplest. As much as ordinary doctors accept patients up to a limit, so disaster caretakers accept patients up to the limit of their professional capacity. By excluding only the mild and the hopeless cases, triage doctors in the clinical scheme avoid potentially regrettable and psychologically excruciating decisions of triage. They do not "play God", but act as humble doctors.

The responsiveness of clinical schemes to the psychological needs of the caring team renders them receptive to "symbolic considerations" as well. Symbolic considerations are defined as narratives that are morally meaningful but clinically neutral. Symbolic-sensitive triage may admit twin brothers, even if one would be rejected by individual evaluation. It may admit a patient because "all of her five brothers and sisters have died" or "because she has miraculously survived under debris for many days". These morally meaningful considerations may not be clinically relevant, let alone dominant. It is quite possible that sensitivity to the moral psychology of the care-givers might be self-defeating as well. Triage by predefined and legitimately accepted rules or set of rules might be much less taxing and may relieve the conscience of the triage person from numerous bio-psycho-social considerations.

One more drawback of the clinical scheme is related to its abhorrence to rejecting patients at the door. This might result in care for the mildly (but not too mildly) injured who manage to arrive before more vulnerable victims such as pregnant women, children, or the non-ambulant. This might be no less psychologically distressing than the very act of rejecting one patient for the sake of anther.

4.3.3 Hybrid Schemes of Triage in Mass Casualty Triage

The third scheme is a utilitarian-clinical hybrid. By observing the traditional divisions separating the clinical sphere from other domains of life, the hybrid scheme refuses to approach each and every medical decision from a purely utilitarian perspective. The hybrid scheme tolerates principled decisions of the kind of care offered in any disaster scenario, whether to send rescue personnel or medical teams, for example. Once a victim is admitted by triage, he or she becomes a patient. From that moment on, the medical team will dedicate efforts to his or her care, not shunning a second or third operation, minding medical complications and co-morbid conditions, not being under pressure to trim care or to discharge prematurely.

Hybrid schemes preserve (at least to a degree) the independence of medical care and the value of fiduciary duties in medical ethics (non-abandonment and continuity of care). The purpose of triage is to fairly select patients who are likely to benefit from the kind of care and expertise available. Triage within hybrid schemes does not aim at selecting the most promising patients, but only patients whose medical needs are urgent enough and of the kind that can be addressed by the team and its resources. Once triage transforms a victim into a patient, care is directed with little regard to the needy victims outside the circle of care. Only minor compromises in the quality of care are permitted for the sake of liberating beds inside the hospital for the sake of new patients.

We contend that the hybrid approach has a practical and a moral justification. The practical justification is best cast in utilitarian terms. Healthcare professionals responsible for triage are not trained in the art of sophisticated prognostications. A body of evidence does not exist to show whether post-amputation care requires two or four days in a field hospital or whether fluids, antibiotics and wound care alone may suffice for a septic burn victim. In the face of such doubts, it is preferable to give the amputee fuller care and not admit the burn patient in her place. Thus, the values of clinical ethics will be preserved, without overt violation of a principled commitment to utility. Put in other words, even in conditions of disaster care, observation of clinical ethics may often promote utility rather than collide with it. Moreover, the hybrid triage suits the clinical setting and the psychological make-up of the healthcare professionals involved. It is especially accommodating of both the clinical bond that is created between caregivers and their patients and the awareness of the special conditions of disaster medicine.

The hybrid scheme is also flexible, allowing different balances between utilitarian or efficiency oriented pressures on the one hand and clinical habits and guidelines on the other.

Table 4.1 shows how different types of patients would be triaged under the three triage schemes. Further practical aspects of using the hybrid scheme are discussed in the remainder of this chapter.

Table. 4.1 How the main triage schemes respond to prototypical patients

Type of patient	Utilitarian	Hybrid	Clinical
No urgent or significant medical need	Reject	Reject	Reject
Low prognosis	Reject	May or may not reject	Admit
Likely to benefit	Admit	Admit	Admit
Likely to benefit but extraordinary burden	Reject	May or may not reject	Admit
Patient may benefit although the team is not equipped to handle her problem	Reject	Reject	Admit
Patient becomes an excessive burden after admittance or becomes needy of unavailable medical attention	Dismiss	Continue care	Continue care
Prognosis deteriorates but care is not futile	Dismiss	Continue care	Continue care
Prognosis deteriorates, care is not futile, but depends on special resource (e.g. ventilation)	Dismiss	Dismiss	Continue care
Early discharge after partial care	Dismiss	Endorse only minor compromise of care	Continue care
Symbolic appeal	Reject	May accept occasionally	Accept

4.3.4 Pre-clinical Triage

An additional consideration looming over all strategies of micro-triage (i.e. the allocation of clinical resources on site) is "pre-clinical triage" whose ethical aspects we do not discuss in this chapter. We define pre-clinical triage as the administrative choices to include or exclude equipment and personnel in humanitarian expeditions. Such decisions depend on the triage strategy chosen. Sometimes, the pre-clinical triage is not flexible (e.g. a military hospital ship may not have certain medical equipment), thus constraining and directing the strategy of triage chosen or some aspects thereof.

Many relief teams that went to Haiti did not bring equipment for the care of neonates and children. The American waterborne hospital that moored offshore refused admittance of paediatric patients. This did not reflect a policy of disaster care, but the simple fact that portable hospitals belong to the military and are designed to care for wounded soldiers. None the less, to the extent to which specific preparations can be made before the dispatch of a humanitarian relief team, pre-clinical triage might have significant impact on clinical triage. In the next section we wish to propose a match between different disasters and the three prototypical triage schemes.

4.3.5 The Relevance of the Triage Schemes in Different Types of Disaster

In the first two paradigmatic cases of disaster, medical care is usually local, or mainly local, and it operates as an arm of a well ordered society. Hence, care is a priori owed to all victims in their capacity as citizens. Caregivers cannot be satisfied with the treatment given to the few while ignoring those selected out during triage. Indeed, many well-ordered societies have detailed laws and ordinances regulating disaster

Table. 4.2 The relative relevance of triage schemes in various disaster circumstances

Disaster prototype		Triage scheme: Utilitarian	Hybrid	Clinical
Ordinary triage	Well circumscribed	Urgency of life-saving medical attention is the sole criteria of care		
Mass-casualty triage	Well circumscribed	Reasonable	Reasonable	Inappropriate
	Disruptive	Most reasonable	Reasonable	Difficult to accept
	Double disaster	Reasonable, although it may verge on the absurd	Reasonable	Most appealing

management and care (Hodge and Anderson 2008). However, in "double disasters" the only moral link between caregivers and victims is the value of human solidarity. Put in other words, the duties of society to its own citizens are of the complete kind, whereas the duty or attitude of solidarity is incomplete. Rejection of victims is more likely to be incompatible in circumstances of complete duty than in circumstances of incomplete duties. Since solidarity is an attitude of the actor, and it does not depend on the outcome of action, it may be argued that solidarity is fulfilled by all three schemes of triage.

This distinction may explain why medical teams may give priority to the medical needs of their own personnel (should somebody get hurt or sick, care for the team member, even if successful, will not restore him or her to beneficial activity). The team owes mutual complete duties of help; the fiduciary duty to other disaster victims comes afterwards.

It seems that the worse the disaster and the more wretched the afflicted society, the more appealing the clinical approach becomes (see Table 4.2). In the face of hundreds of thousands of victims and in the absence of infrastructure, the utilitarian impact of humanitarian expeditions seems negligent. If there is any meaning at all in clinical care, it probably lies in its humane defiance of despair, helplessness and erosion in human dignity. Suppose the utilitarian scheme saves a hundred lives out of ten thousand victims, and the clinical one saves only thirty people. The difference between the two strategies amounts to less than one percent of all people whose lives are at stake. Is such a tiny bit of difference worth the utilitarian degradation of people into objects in a machine of care that keeps rejecting the weakest and trampling on traditional roles, professional boundaries, habits of care and the psychological distress of caretakers? To this question the utilitarian would respond that even if the difference between the utilitarian scheme and its competitors amounts to only one single person saved, a deliberate preference for the non-utilitarian schemes amounts to disrespect for human dignity, as if one single person does not count (Parfit 1978).

In all of the scenarios, the hybrid scheme is responsive to utilitarian considerations, while protecting the clinical sphere from relentless utilitarian pressures that are incompatible with the values of clinical ethics and that might lack firm justification based on medical knowledge. Hybrid schemes do not require healthcare professionals to deviate much from their modes of thought and practice, thus preserving their sense of personal integrity as well as the integrity of medical care.

Awareness of the frustration at keeping a low-prognosis (but never very low) patient in ICU while more promising victims are dying outside, helps us appreciate the importance of triage and that the dominant value during triage is utilitarian beneficence. Accurate choice of patients (by utilitarian standards) is the best guarantee against dilemmas of loyalty such as the one between the septic patient and the new one. It may be observed that it is precisely the wish to preserve some clinical values inside the medical setting that justifies stricter utilitarian considerations at the gate (triage).

4.4 An Outline for a Hybrid Scheme of Triage

For every hypothetical victim of disaster one may project an ideal plan of salvage. This plan is divisible into discrete steps (see Fig. 4.1). Some steps are non-medical (e.g. rescue from under debris, transfer to a medical facility), while others are medical. By definition, triage occurs when a healthcare professional decides whether to make the victim pass from the non-medical stage of rescue into the stage of medical care. In utilitarian and hybrid schemes of care, triage-like decisions also take place during medical care, when things turn to the worse, or when new claimants for care appear at the door.

Triage itself may be conceived as a stage rather than a junction. As a stage, it may benefit from consulting an ad-hoc ethics committee (Merin et al. 2010). During the triage period, victims may receive pain control, basic nursing care (e.g. food, blankets, registration of demographic data), simple but essential care (e.g. fixation of a dislocated jaw, external control of bleeding) and await relevant results (e.g. haemoglobin, myoglobin). The dying may be moved aside to a quiet area and be tended to by non-professional volunteers. Care is expected to be more efficient and more humane when triage is construed as a stage of basic care and not only as a sorting point. In case the medical services are flooded with victims, even this kind of triage may be impossible to achieve. In such circumstances the diagnostic reliability of triage decreases, thus reducing further the reliability and desirability of utilitarian strategies.

Typically, the triage person contemplates four key questions. The first two questions aim at determining the "urgency of need", which according to the World Medical Association (WMA), is the main criterion of triage in disaster care (WMA 2006)). Is the victim in need of medical attention (rather than non-medical assistance such as shelter, psychological support or medical care that is not urgent or indispensable)? Does the victim stand a reasonable chance of medical benefit (rather than being hopeless or in need of unavailable medical means)?

However, the person responsible for triage may contemplate two more questions: Is the victim likely to consume medical resources more than the average patient? Is the team ready to address the victim's main problem (e.g. a team of orthopaedic surgeons may be unsuited to care for a child with second degree burns)?

According to the hybrid scheme, triage aims at selecting victims who are likely to benefit from the clinical competencies of the team. A team of orthopaedic surgeons

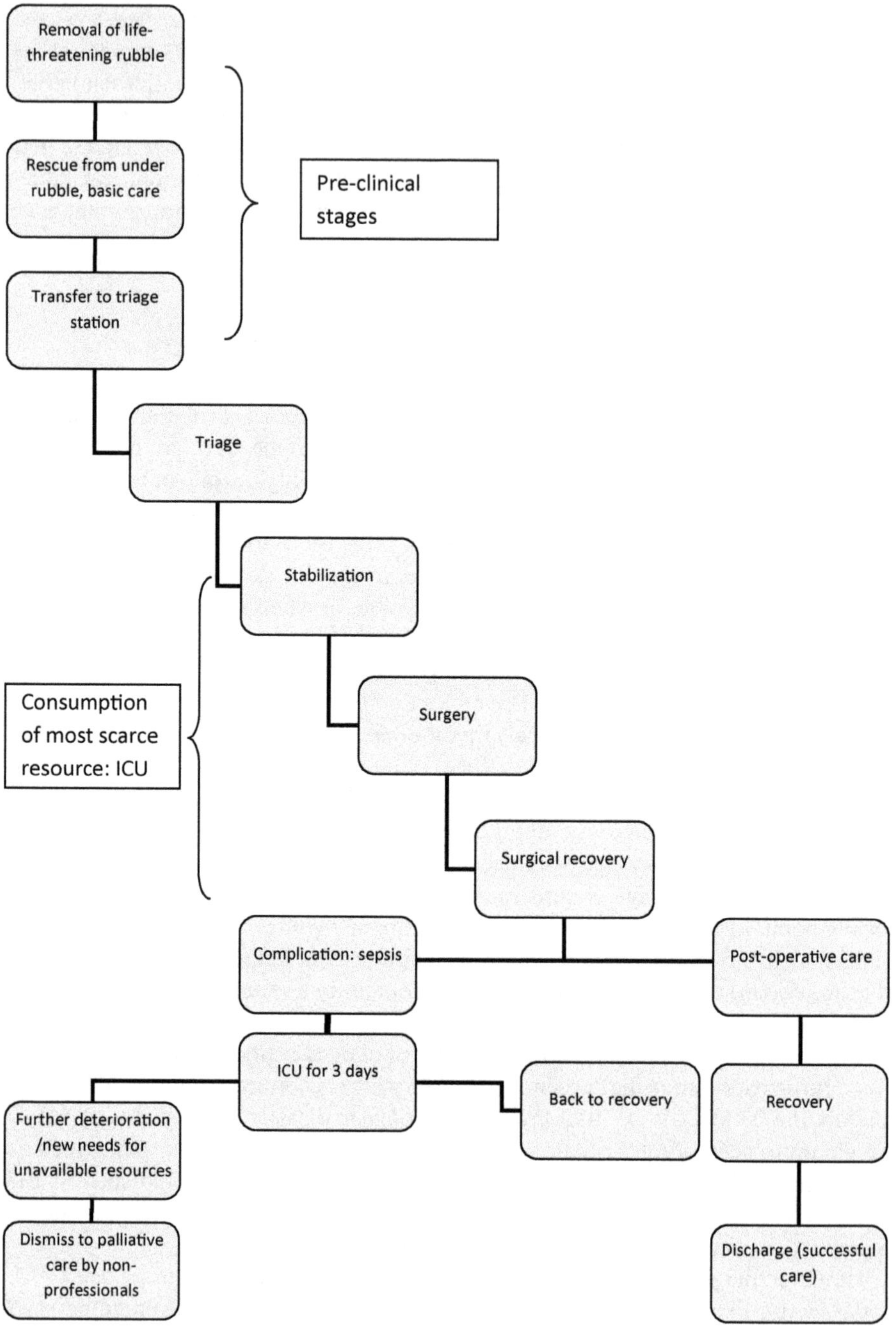

Fig. 4.1 Plan for triage

is likely to select victims with fractures and crush injury. The team may select fracture patients over crush injury patients because more fracture patients are likely to complete all necessary steps towards discharge, while crush injury patients may need dialysis and prolonged mechanical ventilation (not only during the operation). The hybrid scheme would reject patients who are likely to depend on unavailable therapy (dialysis) and preserve the scarce resource (ventilation) for the sake of patients in need of available therapy (fracture care). Ventilation serves the latter during surgery or following complications (sepsis). However, if a fracture patient develops renal failure while already a patient, she will not be dismissed from care. From a utilitarian perspective, her claim to care has become identical to the claim of the rhabdomyolysis patient. In the clinical and hybrid schemes, patients are dismissed only when a stable clinical goal has been achieved or when the team cannot benefit them medically any more. Their next step of care is not weighed against the needs of patients undergoing triage at the door.

Not only utilitarian schemes, but also hybrid schemes of triage depend on good assessment of the disaster overall—estimate of damage, types of injury, other venues of help, and potential risks. Triage decisions about individual patients are not taken with the previous or next victim in mind, but against a general estimate of needs and resources. A decision to admit one patient should not be deliberated on against the story of the previous patient, as if the triage doctor decides to save John and let Mary die. John and Mary are coincidentally presenting themselves to the triage team simultaneously. This coincidence may be a source of cognitive and emotional bias. Triage schemes are guideline-dependent, although the dynamics of disaster care imply frequent reassessment and revision. The specific guidelines of the team are determined ad hoc and are the responsibility of the team. Triage is not a personal decision, although it is executed by healthcare professionals who examine patients.

4.5 Conclusion

In this chapter we have presented three general schemes for triage in disaster. The extremities of disaster and its direct assault on the very basics of human existence and values render the search for one "morally best" strategy of triage futile. With the exception of clearly malicious approaches (e.g. racism), it is also very difficult to dismiss triage policies as immoral. This does not render the search for ethical strategies of triage a useless pursuit. Over and above the wish for acting morally, insight into the nature of events and meaning-giving are at the heart of moral deliberation. They are essential for successful coping (Updegraff et al. 2008). Moreover, these explorations may shed light on urgent issues such as macro-allocation in disaster relief and global justice (see Chapter 2).

The concept of justice has always had two layers of meaning. On the one hand, justice is an agent-relative term; it is the right thing that the person or persons should do. On the other hand, it is a human valuation of states of affairs, regardless of agency. We say that the death of a child is "unjust", even when nothing could be done about it. We need to cultivate awareness of the tragic fact that disasters are states of affairs that are so unjust so as render humanitarian intervention noble and just despite its frustrating finitude.

Bernard Williams explains the controversy between the "realists" and the "non-realists."

> The non-realist approach may allow for the possibility that one can be forced to two inconsistent moral judgments about the same situation, each of them backed by the best possible reasons, and each of them firmly demanding acceptance; and while action or advice demands deciding between them, it does not demand—or permit—deciding that either of them was wrong, or only apparently a requirement of the situation. The inconsistency does not necessarily show that something was wrong—except with the situation. Whereas on the realist view, this just could not ultimately be the state of affairs. (Williams 1973, p. 205)

The realities of disaster are too surreal to allow for a "realist" meta-ethics (see Chapter 3 on non-ideal ethics). We have argued that although different approaches to triage in disaster might produce incompatible moral judgments, they are nevertheless consistent with the best humans can do in such extreme states of affairs.

References

Barilan, Y. M. 2004. Towards a dialogue between utilitarianism and medicine. *Medicine Healthcare and Philosophy* 7:163–173.

Burris, D. G., D. R. Welling, and N. M. Rich. 2004. Dominique Jean Larrey and the principle of humanity in warfare. *Journal of the American College of Surgeons* 198:832–835.

Calabresi, G., and P. Bobbitt. 1978. *Tragic choices: the conflicts society confronts in the allocation of tragically scarce resources*. New York: Norton.

Emanuel, E. J., and A. Wertheimer. 2006. Who should get influenza vaccine when not all can? *Science* 312:854–855.

Fleck, L. 2009. *Just caring: Healthcare rationing and democratic deliberation*. Oxford: Oxford University Press.

Gross, M. 2006. *Bioethics and armed conflict: Moral dilemmas of medicine and war*. Cambridge (MA): MIT Press.

Hodge, J. G., and E. D. Anderson. 2008. Principles and practice of legal triage during public health emergencies. *New York Annual Survey of American Law* 64:249–292.

International Federation of Red Cross. 1995. The code of conduct for the International Red Cross and Red Crescent Movement and non-governmental organisations (NGOs) in disaster relief. http://www.ifrc.org/Docs/idrl/I259EN.pdf. Accessed 6 May 2013.

Iserson, K. V. 2008. Flight or fight: The ethics of emergency physician disaster response. *Annals of Emergency Medicine* 51:345–353.

Iserson, K. V., and N. Pesik. 2003. Ethical resource distribution after biological, chemical or radiological terrorism. *Cambridge Quarterly of Healthcare Ethics* 12:455–465.

Kass, N. E., J. Otto, D. O'Brien, and M. Minson. 2008. Ethics and severe pandemic influenza: Maintaining essential functions through fair and considered response. *Biosecurity and Bioterrorism: Biodefense Strategy, Practice, and Science* 6:227–236.

Mayerfeld, J. 1999. *Suffering and moral responsibility*. Oxford: Oxford University Press.

Merin, O., N. Ash, G. Levy, M. J. Schwaber, and Y. Kreiss. 2010. The Israeli field hospital in Haiti—ethical dilemmas in early disaster response. *New England Journal of Medicine* 362:e38.

Parfit, D. 1978. Innumerate ethics. *Philosophy and Public Affairs* 7:285–301.

Rawls, J. 1971. *A theory of justice*. Cambridge: Harvard University Press.

Sorokin, P. A. 1942. *Man and society in calamity*. New York: Dutton.

Updegraff, J. A., R. Cohen Silver, and E. A. Holman. 2008. Searching for and finding meaning in collective trauma: Results from a national longitudinal study of 9/11 terrorists attacks. *Journal of Personality and Social Psychology* 95:709–722.

White, D. B., M. H. Katz, J. M Luce, and B. Lo. 2009. Who should receive life-support during public health emergency? Using ethical principles to improve allocation decisions. *Annals of Internal Medicine* 150:132–138.

Williams, B. 1973. *Problems of the self.* Cambridge: Cambridge University Press.

Winslow, G. R. 1982. *Triage and justice*. Berkeley: University of California Press.

World Medical Association. 2006. Statement on medical ethics in the event of disasters. http://www.wma.net/en/30publications/10policies/d7/. Accessed 6 May 2013.

Chapter 5
When Relief Comes from a Different Culture: Sri Lanka's Experience of the Asian Tsunami

Athula Sumathipala

5.1 Disasters

According to the Emergency Disasters Database (EM-DAT) there were 16,000 major disasters leading to over 500,000 deaths in the last hundred years. In 2010 alone there were 373 natural disasters, affecting 207 million people and resulting in 296,800 deaths (Lancet 2011). They included the earthquake in Haiti, heat wave in Russia, earthquakes, landslides and floods in China, and the earthquake in Indonesia. In addition, other large scale disasters in the past few years include the tsunami in Sri Lanka, earthquakes in Pakistan, floods in India, Hurricane Katrina in the USA, landslides in the Philippines, typhoon in Myanmar and, most recently, the 2011 Japanese tsunami. These have brought up many novel challenges in the ethics of disaster management.

5.2 Disasters and Ethical Issues in Disasters

Disasters cause destruction, death, disease/disorders, displacement, disappearance, and disarray (the 6 Ds). All of these have implications for ethics and human rights (Sumathipala and Jafarey 2010). The management of all components of the above consequences of disasters has strong ethical implications. "Ethical entry" into disaster-affected communities should be considered a prerequisite by those who are "duty bound" not to add further negative consequences to what is already faced by disaster survivors. According to Citraningtyas and colleagues, 'Ethical entry into a community requires recognition of and mitigation of the potential impacts of entry into a community, for example, culturally and socioeconomically. Ideally, ethical engagement requires an approach beyond community involvement or even community partnership, so that the community holds ownership and leadership of the processes'

A. Sumathipala (✉)
King's College, London, UK
e-mail: athula.sumathipala@kcl.ac.uk

D. P. O'Mathúna et al. (eds.), *Disaster Bioethics: Normative Issues When Nothing is Normal,* Public Health Ethics Analysis 2, DOI 10.1007/978-94-007-3864-5_5,

(Citraningtyas et al. 2010, p. 109). In other words, relief should not be imposed by the donor's will but should be dependent on the needs of the affected community. The authors argue that this is a fundamental moral obligation of those who are involved in disaster relief operations.

The consequences of disasters (the 6 Ds) may be universal, but management of disasters undoubtedly has different perspectives in different cultures, resulting in ethical dilemmas (Harman and Thomson 1996). One good example is how one of the Ds (death) leads to issues around the handling of dead bodies after a disaster. This results in grief, but various people and cultures resolve grief differently. Death and burial are universal activities, but the practice of burial and the rituals involved in funerals vary enormously between cultures and communities. Taking a simple example, Muslim communities around the world would dispose of dead bodies within 24 hours. 'Muslims are always buried, never cremated. It is a religious requirement that the body be ritually washed and draped before burial, which should be as soon as possible after death' (Gatrad 1994, p. 521). Muslim women never attend burials. However this is completely different for those who practice Buddhism. They have a different set of rituals and keep the body for more than a day. They may also cremate the body. Another difference is that Muslims link death to God's will whereas Buddhists would link death to Karma (fate).

5.3 Culture

The purview of this chapter does not allow a detailed discussion of culture. However a brief account will be helpful to place the issues discussed into their context. There are many definitions of culture, which is an abstract concept. However there is some agreement 'that culture is learned and shared, it is dynamic and ever-changing, and it is the way people structure and adapt to their internal and external environments' (Bhugra and Mastrogianni 2004, p. 11). 'It refers to patterns of perceiving and adapting to the world. Culture is reflected in the learned, shared beliefs, values, attitudes and behaviours characteristic of a society or population' (Bhugra and Mastrogianni 2004, p. 11).

As a result, there are 'culturally specific ways of expressing emotional distress and what constitutes appropriate healing. All expressions of emotional distress, including the acute grief of the survivors of this disaster, are embedded within, and cannot be separated from, particular cultural frameworks' (Gilbert 2005, p. 5).

5.3.1 Culture and Language

Language plays a crucial role in culture. Thousands of languages are spoken around the world and determine how people communicate their feelings and perceptions about themselves, others and the world. 'Some of these fundamental concepts are unique to that community's ways of perceiving the world, and cannot be directly translated into another language without serious loss of meaning' (Gilbert 2005, p. 5). Each person experiences and expresses emotions, therefore, within the constraints of a particular language and the culture embedded within it.

5.3.2 Culture, Language and Disasters

Because the 6 Ds are inevitable consequences of disasters, and all have significant emotional impact, all could be manifest in culturally specific ways. These include the language people speak and behaviours linked to their shared beliefs, values, and attitudes. Therefore the 'culture' of a disaster-affected community, the way the people think, feel and behave in relation to coping, should be respected by those who come from a different culture to offer help. Collective belief systems should not be ignored by those who may not necessarily agree with them or even be unfamiliar with them just because they come from a completely different culture.

Religion is an important component of a culture. The issue of religion and culture therefore plays an important role during disaster response. This topic would require a chapter in itself, but it is worth noting that some might see any disaster as the 'will of the gods' and something supernatural to be accepted. Others would turn to god to battle against the disaster as a natural phenomenon, and then non-religious people might be disparaging of any religious view.

5.4 International Assistance and Relief in Disasters

International assistance following disasters may come from Non-Governmental Organisations (NGOs), International NGOs (INGOs) or individuals, including expatriates. These efforts may be purely philanthropic, which is 'the effort or inclination to increase the well-being of humankind, as by charitable aid or donations' (Ahmad and Mahmud 2010, p.154). At the same time, assistance could also be influenced by other factors that create conflicts of interest (Sumathipala and Siribaddana 2005). For example, when humanitarian aid comes from agencies or individuals who may also conduct or sponsor research projects, there will be implicit conflicts of interest leading to philanthropic misconception (Ahmad and Mahmud 2010). However this is only one form of conflict of interest among many.

In this chapter, the Sri Lankan post-tsunami experience will be revisited to examine the issues that surfaced in relation to cultural issues and the resulting ethical issues that arose when relief came from a different culture. This is particularly important as many issues, including management of the dead, are culture-specific. Even universal needs, like that for shelter, have a cultural component. For example, while everyone needs shelter from the elements, the extent to which privacy is important will vary by culture. Within Sri Lanka, while Western medical relief is generally acceptable, in some parts of the country people will be drawn to traditional healers and this needs to be taken into account.

5.4.1 The Tsunami

On 26 December 2004, an earthquake with a magnitude of 9.3 occurred resulting in the catastrophic tsunami which affected 12 countries (Kruger and Ohrnberger 2005; Lay et al. 2005). Four countries (Indonesia, Sri Lanka, India and Thailand) were worst affected (Ng 2005). The human impact of this tsunami was enormous in terms of individuals and families affected, displaced or killed. More than 200,000 people were killed (Ng 2005). Almost 2 million lost their homes and had to find shelter with family, friends or in temporary settlements.

About one third of Sri Lanka was affected. The estimated death toll in Sri Lanka alone was more than 30,000; many more thousands of people went missing and were displaced. Hundreds of Western holiday-makers became its victims, along with local hotel staff (Watters 2010).

5.4.2 Sri Lanka

Sri Lanka has a population of 20 million. It is a multi-ethnic society where the majority (74 %) is Sinhalese while 18 % are Tamil and 7 % Moor. The remaining 1 % consists of Burgher, Malay and Veddas. Seventy percent of the population is Buddhist. The remaining are Hindus (15 %), Christians (8 %) and Muslims (7 %). Vital statistics are amongst the best in South Asia, with the literacy rate over 92.5 % in males and 87.9 % in females and life expectancy averages 74 years in males and females. Crude death rate is 5.9 per 1,000 population and the maternal mortality rate is 3.5 per 10,000 live births. Infant mortality is 15.4 per 1,000 live births (Ministry of Health 2005). Sri Lanka has an extensive public health network and health services are provided free to the public. On the other hand, Sri Lanka has witnessed 30 years of internal conflicts, political violence, and has high alcohol consumption per person and a high suicide rate compared to other countries (Eddleston et al. 1998; Samarasingha et al. 1987).

5.4.3 Strengths

The most significant strength in Sri Lanka was social cohesion; people, even in the directly affected areas, were supporting one another in the immediate aftermath of the tsunami. There was voluntary participation and contribution from people throughout the country. Within 24 h of the disaster, essential items were pouring into affected areas from non-affected areas. Even in the Northern and Eastern parts of Sri Lanka, which were affected at that time by separatist terrorism, people were permitted to come from other parts to provide relief. There were contributions from the public, political parties, local NGOs and INGOs. The displaced people were accommodated in shelters provided by temples, schools, friends and relatives in the first 24 h (WHO

2005a). Statutory services were involved to restore the basic needs. Restoration of electricity and water, and clearance of roads and towns, started within four days.

While Sri Lanka was not prepared for a disaster of this scale, a large number of statutory organisations did what they ought to do in a disaster situation, even though the response was fragmented and uncoordinated during the initial few days. Human resources were plentiful.

5.4.4 *Governmental Response*

Within the first 48 hours of the tsunami, the government established a Centre for National Operations (CNO) to coordinate both national and international relief operations as a temporary crisis intervention centre. The CNO provided the essential interface between concerned government ministries, local authorities, the military, and the international community (Sumathipala and Siribaddana 2005). The author, who was doing full time research in Sri Lanka at the time, was invited to lead the psychosocial section at the CNO.

5.4.5 *Cultural Mismatch*

A unique feature of the Asian tsunami was the scale of the global public reaction it attracted. Other recent disasters may have claimed more lives, but none has triggered such a massive international response. Soon after the tsunami over $7 billion was pledged (BBC 2005; see Table 5.1.).

Countries in the region (India, Bangladesh and Afghanistan) also offered indirect non-financial help. Two months after the tsunami, $40 million in aid to Sri Lanka had been received by the Central Bank of Sri Lanka. Meanwhile, private NGOs had received $600 million (Yamada et al. 2006).

However there were significant cultural mismatches arising from the 'humanitarian assistance' pouring in following the tsunami. Tensions arose from diverse models utilised in the management of potential psychological consequences of trauma, management of the dead bodies, international groups rushing in with 'aids', making the survivors dependent rather than empowering them, exploitation of the vulnerable survivors for easy and cheap research, and many other unethical practices. These issues will be discussed later in this chapter.

5.4.6 *The Second Wave of Tsunami*

Immediately after the tsunami, numerous NGOs arrived from abroad in Sri Lanka and started work, but with lots of duplication creating significant coordination problems. The author, as the coordinator of the psychosocial section of the CNO, personally witnessed these hardships. Large numbers of NGOs from foreign countries

Table 5.1 Donations pledged or provided

Country	Amount of donation pledged or provided
Japan	$500 m (£264 m) in government donations; $70 m had been allocated to UNICEF and $60 m to the UN World Food Programme
United States	$350 m in government donations, and around $200 m in private donations, with $120 m donated to the US branches of the Red Cross, Oxfam and Save the Children, and to Catholic Relief Services
Norway	$183 m in government donations, plus an estimated $30 m raised in private donations
Britain	$96 m in government donations, plus an estimated $466 m in private donations which the government pledged to match
Italy	$95 m in government aid. Public donations totalling $20 m had been collected by New Year's Day
Sweden	$80 m in government donations, of which around $20 m has been disbursed, plus at least $75 m in private donations
Denmark	$75 m in government aid
Spain	$68 m in government donations
France	$66 m in government donations, plus an estimated $90 m raised in private
Canada	$343 m in government donations, plus at least $75 m raised in private donations
China	$83 m in government donations, plus $1.8 m donated to the Chinese Red Cross
Australia	The Government raised its offer of aid to $764 m over five years
Netherlands	$34 m has been donated by the government as emergency aid. A further $259 m has been allocated for reconstruction. Aid groups say a further $35 m has been raised in private donations
Russia	Around $10 m in government aid to be distributed over the first half of the year
Germany	Government aid of $647 m over three years. The public have donated an estimated $586 m
Qatar	$25 m in government aid. Qatar is also sending food, medical and logistical supplies to affected countries
World Bank	$250 m diverted from existing programs to cover emergency needs while longer-term reconstruction needs are assessed.
European Union	$628 m in reconstruction and humanitarian funds, of which $130 m is humanitarian aid. (The total sum donated by the EU and its member States was roughly $2 bn.)
International Monetary Fund (IMF)	Up to $1bn offered to afflicted countries. The IMF also extended the schedule of Sri Lanka's debt repayments, which will reduce interest payments by about $114 m in 2011
Asian Development Bank	$500 m has been allocated to Indonesia, Sri Lanka and the Maldives in the form of grants and highly concessional funds. The bank says up to $175 m more could be diverted from on-going programs

wanted to provide counselling. However some of the groups did not have people who could communicate in English which is spoken by a fair percentage of Sri Lankans. Finding appropriate translators was an additional burden. Similarly there were many groups wanting to provide medical aid which was already adequately available within the country from areas not impacted by the tsunami. The effectiveness of the activities carried out by those coming from abroad was limited because they lacked knowledge of local languages, culture, health infrastructure and epidemiology (WHO 2005a). They encountered linguistic and cultural barriers. These barriers were especially notable in the care of patients with psychiatric symptoms, for whom diagnosis and treatment is dependent on effective, culturally competent, history taking (Sumathipala et al. 2006).

5.4.6.1 Psychological Support

One of the glaring issues was lack of familiarity with the remarkable psychological resilience of Sri Lankan people. In spite of three decades of war, armed uprising and conflict, communities have remaining functional and hopeful (Fernando 2005). Medicalization of distress, and assumptions about Western models of illness and healing applying in other cultural settings, were major issues (Watters 2010). Some responders advocated a strict Post-Traumatic Stress model in which denial of traumatic stress is seen as a profound error which will lead to much preventable suffering (Watters 2010). However, there is a wider agreement that single one-off compulsory debriefing of trauma victims is harmful (Yamada et al. 2006). The World Health Organisation believes that the threat posed by post-traumatic stress disorder is overstated and focus should be on the recognition and treatment of common mental disorders (Rose et al. 2002).

Although there were clear signs that people were coping well with this disaster, certain NGOs and individuals advocated and offered inappropriate psychological and social support, ignoring traditional social support systems in the country (Watters 2010). 'Hundreds of nongovernmental organisations, universities and private groups quickly began to gather resources and make plans to send an army of trauma counsellors' from the USA, Australia, New Zealand, UK and France (Watters 2010, p. 70). One group came to the author wanting to provide counselling services but did not speak English, only French. Another overseas group came to train people to do Eye Movement Desensitisation and Reprocessing (EMDR)—a technique that needs a high degree of training and skills (Shapiro 2001).[1] Strangely a group from abroad decided to train a group of cricket umpires in the technique.

Watters describes in detail how the trauma counselling was imposed on a completely different culture where people had their own ways of coping, where psychological support came naturally through their own traditional mechanisms that had been in place for hundreds of years (Watters 2010). 'The idea that people from different cultures might have fundamentally different psychological reactions to a traumatic event' is hard for some to grasp (Watters 2010, p. 71).

Interestingly, a recently concluded study revealed that the demand for such services was extremely low, as people who sought external help were more interested

---

[1] EMDR is a form of psychotherapy that was developed by Francine Shapiro to resolve the development of trauma-related disorders caused by exposure to distressing events.

in getting support from traditional healers or traditional physicians, which included astrologers, diviners, oracles and traditional doctors (especially Ayurvedic doctors) (Ekanayake 2010, Ekanayake et al. 2013). This study also revealed that 'survivors' accounts indicate that many were able to draw on resiliencies rooted in religious faith and practices, and cultural traditions to sustain their emotional well-being. Support from family and friends, outside organizations, community members or professionals were identified as the important sources of help' (Ekanayake 2010, p. 266). This in-depth qualitative study also revealed that 'many women and older participants, reiterating the importance and relevance of their faith and religion and to make sense of their losses; tsunami was an example of Buddha's preaching on tentativeness in life and nature. Many Buddhists believed that they escaped from death or other hardships due to previous merits and "good Karma"' (Ekanayake 2010, p. 180). 'The Catholic and Muslim participants were also convinced that God had helped them to escape from such a catastrophe ("it was God's will") and that God would protect them from any future disaster' (Ekanayake et al. 2013, p. 71). They found that engagement in religious activities increased during the early days after the tsunami; visits to religious places, talking to priests and praying or using prayer beads were increased by Catholics in the study sample. Similarly, Muslim participants had more frequent visits to mosques and greater adherence to the practice of praying five times a day (Ekanayake 2010, p. 216).

The need for counselling was overstated because of predicted prevalence rates for conditions like post-traumatic stress disorder and depression that were 'between 50 and 90 percent of the affected population' (Watters 2010, p. 69). Contrary to those assumptions, the National Mental Health Survey commissioned by the Ministry of Health in Sri Lanka, conducted by the Institute for Research and Development and led by the author, revealed in 2007 that the overall PTSD rate for Sri Lanka was only 1.7 %, much lower than the predicted rates. Even in the directly affected tsunami regions and areas affected by war the rate was 2.4 %. Major depression was only 2 %. Emotional or conduct disorders among children were also found not to be significantly more prevalent in tsunami-affected areas compared to areas not affected (Institute for Research and Development 2007).

5.4.6.2 Pharmaceuticals

Considering other interventions, some groups who came from abroad provided survivors with cholera vaccination or anti-malarial prophylaxis. However, this was not appropriate as the threat of cholera was negligible due to the excellent public health infrastructure in Sri Lanka and the coastal region being non-endemic for malaria. Appropriately, the epidemiology unit vaccinated all survivors with measles and gave Vitamin A megadoses to children. In contrast, some donated pharmaceuticals were expired and brands unfamiliar (Sumathipala et al. 2006). Some of these stocks were either outdated when delivered, or became outdated soon after their delivery or before their probable use. Other products were delivered for which there is no use, some were labelled in foreign languages that could not be understood by local staff, and some products were not registered in Sri Lanka. Some products were supplied in quantities that would meet the needs of the whole local population for ten years. Other donations of questionable value included winter jackets, expired cans of food, stiletto shoes, winter tents, thong panties and Viagra.

5.4.7 Work Related to Children and the Education Sector

Children were encouraged to express their emotions by providing them with drawing material (The Island 2005). Early reopening of schools was advocated, as the usual practice in a disaster was to take over schools as temporary shelters. The aim was to get children back to school with dignity. This approach was advocated by education authorities and the Centre for National Operations. However these efforts were criticised by some NGOs and individuals who came from abroad. Watters described one trauma counselor who worried that 'the local children appeared more interested in returning to school than discussing their experience of the tsunami' (Watters 2010, p. 77). This counsellor claimed these children were 'clearly in denial', and that later they would 'experience the full emotional horror of what has happened to them' (Watters 2010, p. 77). However, this reflected a very different view of children and their role in society than exists in Sri Lanka.

5.4.8 Dead Bodies and Forensic Work

Identification of dead bodies is important to allow a dignified burial and is crucial to alleviate long-term psychological and legal consequences (WHO 2005b). Immediately after the tsunami, dead bodies were disposed of rapidly based on the myth (held both locally and by international relief workers) that corpses pose a high risk for epidemics (Sumathipala et al. 2006). This was inappropriate in the context of cultural norms and the potential harmful psychological impact on survivors of non-identification of dead bodies (WHO 2005b). A few Western governments desecrated mass graves to identify their own nationals using DNA techniques without offering these services to the local people (Sumathipala and Siribaddana 2005).

5.5 Post Tsunami Campaign on Ethics

The tsunami was followed by a huge influx of foreign organisations and individuals. When research is combined with humanitarian aid and clinical care, there can be undue inducement on a vulnerable population to participate in research (Sumathipala and Siribaddana 2005). Issues get more complicated because researchers might rush to collect data, without adequate planning and under the guise of "needs assessments" (Sumathipala and Siribaddana 2005). Research can include clinical care but this should be made explicit to participants because while clinical care is routine, research is not, particularly when conducted in the developing world. Otherwise, survivors are at risk of exploitation by research disguised as clinical care, leading to the therapeutic misconception (Martin 2005). Many tsunami survivors were not made clearly aware that they were participating is research.

A classic example involved investigators from a renowned university in a developed country in Asia who were collecting blood samples from tsunami survivors living in temporary shelters in the Southern Province of Sri Lanka (Siribaddana et al. 2010). This example was also brought to the attention of the author in his capacity as the Coordinator for the psychosocial section of the Centre for National Operations established by the Government following the Tsunami. It was reported by the Regional Epidemiologist.

This research took place initially without local ethics clearance but later the investigators identified a local collaborator and an institution (an NGO) and applied for ethical approval from an Ethics Review Committee (ERC) in a prestigious Sri Lankan university. The founder and head of this NGO was the chair of this ERC and a close relative of the local collaborator. They were granted ethical clearance after an expedited review (Siribaddana et al. 2010).

This particular case became widely known and has been subjected to discussion at international conferences (Siribaddana et al. 2010). Knowing that there are likely to be many international academics who would want to undertake evaluations and research after disasters, an awareness raising conference was held on the ethics of research in post-disaster situations led by the Institution for Research and Development (Siriwardana 2007). A significant amount of follow-up work took place to develop disaster research-related ethics guidelines (Sumathipala et al. 2010). These are discussed further in Chapter 7 of this volume.

5.5.1 The Way Forward

The following is an excellent summary of an appropriate mind-set for those entering other cultures to ensure local people are treated with respect.

> Remember you are a "guest" in the country and are there to help local people to help themselves, not to create dependency. Treat all with dignity, especially the dead, who may have died without it. Aim to foster cooperation and the restoration of motivation, self belief, and self sufficiency. (Palmer 2005, p. 152)

There are many important lessons to be learned by 'international communities'. Taking the Sri Lankan tsunami experience, a country where the education and health services were free and strong, the potential for undermining these services was the biggest threat. Secondly, unscrupulous researchers exploited vulnerable survivors. The traumatised should not be re-traumatised by unethical research done without respect for vulnerable survivors for easy and cheap research. Tensions arose from the failure to recognise the complementary nature of different models to address psychological issues. Some stakeholders rigidly argued for a psychosocial model which called for counselling for each and every person, while others were adamant about the medical model where services were to be provided in hospitals and clinics.

In the future all stakeholders should respect the consensus that compulsory counselling should not be done as it could even be counterproductive and harmful. It is important to understand and value the cultural and traditional coping mechanisms and resources available in local settings, particularly before providing psychological treatments to non-Western disaster survivors

References

Ahmad, A, and S. M. Mahmud. 2010. Philanthropic misconception. *Asian Bioethics Review* 2 (2): 154–161.

BBC. 2005. Tsunami aid: Who's giving what. BBC News, 27 January. http://news.bbc.co.uk/1/hi/world/asia-pacific/4145259.stm. Accessed 1 Oct 2011.

Bhugra, D. and Mastrogianni, A. 2004. Globalisation and mental disorders: Overview with relation to depression. *British Journal of Psychiatry* 184 (1): 10–20.

Citraningtyas, T., E. McDonalds, and H. Herman. 2010. A second tsunami? The ethics of coming into communities following disaster. *Asian Bioethics Review* 2 (2): 108–123.

Eddleston, M, R. Sheriff, and K. Hawton. 1998. Deliberate self-harm in Sri Lanka: An overlooked tragedy in the developing world. *British Medical Journal* 317:133–135.

Ekanayake, S. 2010. A qualitative study of psychosocial consequences and coping strategies among tsunami survivors in Sri Lanka. PhD thesis King's College London.

Ekanayake, S., M. Prince, A. Sumathipala, S. Siribaddana, and C. Morgan. 2013. We lost all we had in a second: Coping with grief and loss after a natural disaster. *World Psychiatry* 12:69–75.

Fernando, A. G. 2005. Interventions for survivors of the tsunami disaster: Report from Sri Lanka. *Journal of Traumatic Stress* 18:267–268.

Gatrad, A. R. 1994. Muslim customs surrounding death, bereavement, postmortem examinations, and organ transplants. *British Medical Journal* 309:521–523.

Gilbert, J. 2005. International responses to the psychological aftermath of the tsunami disaster: A plea for thoughtfulness and care. *Counselling and Psychotherapy Journal* 16 (1): 5–6.

Harman, G., and J. J. Thomson. 1996. *Moral relativism and moral objectivity*. Oxford: Blackwell.

Institute for Research and Development (IRD). 2007. National Mental Health Survey in Sri Lanka. Colombo, Sri Lanka.

Kruger, F., and M. Ohrnberger. 2005. Tracking the rupture of the M_W = 9.3 Sumatra earthquake over 1,150 km at teleseismic distance. *Nature* 16:937–939.

Lancet. 2011. Natural disasters—taking a longer term view. *Lancet* 377:439.

Lay, T., H. Kanamori, C. J. Ammon, M. Nettles, S. N. Ward, R. C. Aster, S. L. Beck, S. L. Bilek, M. R. Brudzinski, R. Butler, H. R. DeShon, G. Ekström, K. Satake, and S. Sipkin. 2005. The great Sumatra-Andaman earthquake of 26 December 2004. *Science* 308:1127–1133.

Martin, R. 2005. Undue inducement in clinical research. *Lancet* 366:275–276.

Ministry of Health. 2005. Ministry of Health Annual Health Bulletin. Colombo, Sri Lanka.

Ng, B. Y. 2005. Grief revisited. *Annals of the Academy of Medicine, Singapore* 34:352–355.

Palmer, I. 2005. Humanitarian aid. Psychological aspects of providing medical humanitarian aid. *British Medical Journal* 331:152–154.

Rose, S., J. Bisson, R. Churchill, and S. Wessely. 2002. Psychological debriefing for preventing post traumatic stress disorder (PTSD). *Cochrane Database of Systematic Reviews*, Issue 2. doi:10.1002/14651858.CD000560.

Samarasingha, D., S. A. W. Dissanayake, and C. P. Wijesingha. 1987. Alcoholism in Sri Lanka: An epidemiological survey. *British Journal of Addiction* 82:1149–1153.

Shapiro, F. 2001. *EMDR: Eye movement desensitization of reprocessing: basic principles, protocols and procedures*, 2nd ed. New York: Guilford Press.
Siribaddana, S., B. Fernando, and R. Goonertne. 2010. Neurobiological stress markers in tsunami survivors: A commentary. *Asian Bioethics Review* 2:162–166.
Siriwardana, C. 2007. Disaster research ethics: A luxury or a necessity for developing countries? Asian Tribune, 13 February. http://www.asiantribune.com/index.php?q=node/4524. Accessed 13 Feb 2013.
Sumathipala, A., and A. Jafarey. 2010. Ethics of disaster management, clinical care and research. *Asian Bioethics Review* 2:105–107.
Sumathipala, A., and S. Siribaddana. 2005. Research and clinical ethics after the tsunami: Sri Lanka. *Lancet* 366:1418–1420.
Sumathipala, A., S. Siribaddana, and C. Perera. 2006. Identification and management of dead bodies as a component of psychosocial interventions after the Tsunami: A view from Sri Lanka. *Intentional Review in Psychiatry* 18:249–253.
Sumathipala, A., A. Jafarey, L. D. de Castro, A. Ahmad, D. Marcer, S. Srinivasan, N. Kumar, S. Siribaddana, S. Sutaryo, A. Bhan, D. Waidyaratne, S. Beneragama, C. Jayasekera, S. Edirisingha, and C. Siriwardhana. 2010. Ethical issues in post-disaster clinical interventions and research: A developing world perspective. Key findings from a drafting and consensus generation meeting of the Working Group on Disaster Research and Ethics (WGDRE) 2007. *Asian Bioethics Review* 2:124–142.
The Island. 2005. The Island online edition, 5 January. http://www.island.lk/2005/01/05/. Accessed 1 May 2011.
Watters, E. 2010. *Crazy like us: The globalization of the American psyche*. New York: Free Press.
World Health Organisation (WHO). 2005a. *Mental health and psychosocial relief efforts after the tsunami in Southeast Asia*. New Delhi: WHO.
World Health Organisation (WHO). 2005b. *Psychosocial care of tsunami-affected populations. Manual for community-level workers*. New Delhi: WHO.
Yamada, S., R. P. Gunatilake, T. M. Roytman, S. Gunatilake, T. Fernando, and L. Fernando. 2006. The Sri Lanka tsunami experience. *Disaster Management & Response* 4:38–48.

Chapter 6
Ethical Issues in Health Communications: Strategies for the (Inevitable) Next Pandemic

Joseph Scanlon

6.1 Introduction

During the late winter and early spring of 1889 a disease outbreak occurred in the town of Fingal in Southwestern Ontario. The local physician diagnosed it as chicken pox. The couple who ran the stage coach from Fingal to Shedden thought he was wrong—both had smallpox as children and believed it was smallpox. They went to the newspaper in nearby St. Thomas and it convinced another physician to examine the situation. He concluded the couple was correct and informed the Southwold Township Board of Health.

Homes with cases of smallpox were quarantined. Schools were shut. Churches were closed. The dead were buried quickly and their clothes burned. Sanitary police blocked roads into St. Thomas and the town constructed its first isolation hospital conveniently close to the cemetery. (St. Thomas used the location again during the flu pandemic in 1918–20.) All this was reported in the local newspaper. For some, it was too late: there were 35 cases of smallpox and 16 deaths (Sims 1984).

Fingal illustrates the problems of dealing with a contagious disease. It must be identified and its nature and seriousness determined. The source must be found and the spread of the disease, if possible, controlled; but both can be difficult. That makes it all the more important that the public is informed of the threat and the actions being taken to deal with it—as happened in 1889.

Communications have expanded since then—there are now radio and television, the internet and social media—and a pandemic is much more serious than a local outbreak. People are also more mobile and a warning may no longer involve only those nearby. Nevertheless, the principles for effective communication in health emergencies are the same: there is still the need for identification, response and communication, and there are still many of the same ethical issues. But there is also a lot of knowledge and experience in dealing with such problems and the advice is

J. Scanlon (✉)
Carleton University, Ottawa, Canada
e-mail: jscanlon@connect.carleton.ca

D. P. O'Mathúna et al. (eds.), *Disaster Bioethics: Normative Issues When Nothing is Normal,* Public Health Ethics Analysis 2, DOI 10.1007/978-94-007-3864-5_6,

consistent: while there may be ways to improve how information is given out, there is no disagreement that communications during a pandemic should be open, complete and as immediate as possible.

6.2 Other Incidents

The Fingal incident occurred more than a century ago but there are recent examples of problems in communication during health emergencies. SARS was not immediately identified nor was its seriousness. Some treating the sick became victims, in one case with fatal consequences. There was public confusion about the threat. In Toronto, persons called a hot line asking if they should be concerned about Chinese neighbours; there was a 'precipitous fall in business for Chinese enterprises, especially restaurants' and there was also an impact on tourism (Joint Pandemic Working Group, p. 6). The message had not sunk in—the threat was not from Chinese people, but from travellers.

During the 2009 H1N1 outbreak there was a problem advising the public about the availability of a vaccine and who should get priority access. Health authorities convinced the public that vaccinations were required but could not meet the resulting demand. There may also be questions about safety. There is always a chance—as the US discovered in 1976—that a new vaccine may have side effects. After a new strain of swine flu was detected at Fort Dix, New Jersey, the President announced a plan to inoculate everyone in the USA:

> The [vaccination] campaign was halted after an association was detected between receiving the vaccine and an increase of an obscure neurological disease known as Guillain-Barre Syndrome. Recriminations followed . . . with the popular perception being that the program was a 'fiasco'. . . several . . . in the programme lost their jobs . . . (Dehner 2007, p. 717)

There were also problems during the anthrax attacks shortly after 9/11:

> Public health officials . . . struggled to provide sufficient precise information about the symptoms of inhalation anthrax to allow the lay public to assess whether they needed to seek medical attention. This problem was compounded by the similarity of symptoms to other common respiratory illnesses. (Reynolds and Seeger 2005, p. 50)

These incidents show there are many reasons why communication about a health emergency is not easy. The fact that there is a threat may not be known for some time. It may take more time for it to be properly identified. (Both issues arose with H1N1 in 2009.) The precise symptoms may not be known. Its seriousness may be difficult to assess. It may be difficult to determine when a vaccine will be available and its allocation may create controversy. It may not be certain the vaccine is entirely safe.

Then there are the ethical questions. Should all information about a threat be released? At what point? What about naming a disease carrier? Is this a violation of personal privacy and is it justified when public safety is involved? What about volunteers? How much do they need to be told about the risks involved? Are they entitled to medical information? Is a vaccine entirely safe? Do the risks involved in using it need to be disclosed? There are even ethical issues about ethical behaviour. Recent research suggests some health care workers may refuse to report for work during a pandemic or may refuse to treat those who are ill. Should this be disclosed? Would disclosure lead to panic?

This chapter describes the issues that must be dealt with in developing a communications strategy for a pandemic. It starts by covering planning and training and the four key criteria: effective communications should not be ad hoc but result from planning; health emergencies cannot be handled solely by the health community; most elements of crisis communications can be anticipated; and there are some basic principles:

- Effective warnings must come from all possible sources, must be delivered by persons with credibility and messages must be consistent and repeated: it takes time and repetition for messages to sink in.
- Communications must be accurate, positive and show concern and empathy. (Being positive means telling people what they can do rather than what they should not do.)
- While news media are important, information can be delivered to a mass audience in many ways including social media—and information released to the media must be released through various other channels to be effective.

It is also important that messages be adjusted or tailored to specific groups and issued in all relevant languages. During the 1918 pandemic the US Public Health Service worked very hard to keep the public informed. In New York City, where there were large Jewish and Italian populations officials took cultural differences into account when they placed messages in the Yiddish newspaper, *Forverts*, or the Italian newspaper, *Il Progresso*. When necessary those papers also scotched rumours (Kraul 2010, p. 123).

It then moves on to ethical concerns. What sort of information needs to be provided if there is a perception of a threat? How should a limited supply of vaccine be allocated and how should that be explained? How appropriate is it to stigmatise individuals by naming them or placarding their homes? Does a concern about public safety override personal privacy? What information must be communicated to persons who are being asked to volunteer? What if medical personnel refuse to treat flu victims?

6.3 Principles of Effective Communication

6.3.1 Planning

The first step towards effective pandemic communications is creating a plan. If it is assumed some victims will be quarantined at home, then it is necessary to decide how quarantine decisions will be made, enforced and communicated to those involved and to the public. It is also necessary to decide how those quarantined will be cared for.

Who will check on them? Who will provide medicine, food and other necessities? If, in contrast, it is assumed that all those ill will need hospital care, plans must be made to open and staff emergency hospitals. In both cases, there will be a need to recruit and train volunteers and that means deciding how to advise potential volunteers about the risks. In short, whether people remain at home or are taken to health care facilities, decisions about what should be done lead to a need for communications; so communications planning is an integral part of all planning.

While it may sound reasonable to assume that communications can be done through news releases and news conferences, persons with specific questions will want to talk to someone. This means keeping the medical community informed. It means establishing and staffing call centres. Call centres are not just for answering questions: first they receive and answer queries, second they note what topics are being raised so that those in charge can be informed. This was done by the Regional Municipality of Ottawa-Carleton during the 1998 ice storm and was exceptionally useful. As issues were raised by callers, the Emergency Operation Centre (EOC) was informed and the issues were covered at the next news conference. Such centres can be extremely busy. Toronto's call centres handled 300,000 calls during SARS, 47,567 of them coming on the peak day. There is no need to staff such centres with medically-trained personnel: most queries can be handled by clerical staff, provided they have ready access to more knowledgeable persons when asked a question they can't answer.

During the 1918–20 influenza pandemic many communities ordered schools, churches, theatres, movie theatres, pool halls and other public facilities closed. One town restricted access to homes where someone had died. Good planning will determine how these decisions will be communicated to those directly affected—those who run schools, churches, etc.—and those indirectly affected—such as teachers, school children and the public.

It is important that decisions are made for handling the dead: how will bodies be recovered from private dwellings? What restrictions will be put on visits to funeral homes? Will places of worship be closed? Will burials be speeded up? What about cremation? Everyone must be told bodies do not pose a threat but that public gatherings for funerals, visitations, or memorial services can spread disease among attendees. It is often assumed the medical examiner or coroner will be involved. In fact if cause of death and the victim's identity is known, there will be little need for that. A decision will also have to be made about whether names of those who die and their cause of death will be announced. After 9/11 and the 2004 Indian Ocean tsunami, some countries, including Canada, would not release information about persons missing and possibly dead because of privacy legislation.

6.3.2 Message Content

There are certain basic elements that need to be covered in public communications. The first is the threat, its seriousness and how it can be recognised. Can it, for example, be distinguished from other diseases that may be present? If so what are the distinct symptoms? How does it spread? Are any sets of the population at greater risk? Second, there is the advice for individuals. What precautions should someone take? Should high risk groups take any special precautions? Is there any vaccine or other medicine available? If so how does someone obtain it? How serious is it? Are there likely to be deaths? The World Health Organization says:

> The public is entitled to information that affects their health and the health of their families.... Communication about personal preventative measures is particularly useful as it empowers the public to take some responsibility for their own health. (World Health Organization 2005, p. 6)

Third, there are questions about what to do if someone becomes ill. How should the sick be treated? What precautions should those looking after them take? Should the sick person be taken to hospital? Where can someone looking after a sick person go for further information? Can someone get assistance to care for a sick person at home? What should be done if someone dies?

Fourth, there are questions about the community generally. What precautions is the community taking? What decisions are being made? Closure of schools, churches? Quarantine of individual homes? Restrictions on attendance at funerals? If a vaccine is available, is it being given on a priority basis? What are those priorities? If a vaccine is not available is one being developed? When is it likely to be available? There may be questions about volunteering. Is there anything an individual or a group or business can do? If someone wants to help where do they go? What skills are needed, required? All these questions can be anticipated and answers worked out in advance. Even if circumstances change, the ability to make decisions is enhanced if options were considered.

6.3.3 Tenor of Message

Messages must be consistent. Advice to medical professionals—which inevitably will be passed on to patients—must be identical to statements being released for public consumption otherwise there will be a reaction both from the public and the media. Such statements also need to be accurate and complete stating what is known.

> Effective crisis communicators are honest, candid and open in their public communication. Such honesty, in the long run, fosters credibility with both the media and the public. Moreover a response that is less than honest may, ultimately, create the perception of wrongdoing.... When communicating with the media organizations should avoid inconsistency by accepting uncertainty and avoid any temptation to offer overly reassuring messages. (Seeger 2006, p. 239–240)

Because pandemics cannot be controlled, because some persons will become very ill and others die, those issuing messages—especially those communicating them in person—should display concern and empathy. In describing the availability of a vaccine, for example, it would be wise to say that the goal is to vaccinate everyone when sufficient vaccine is available but that while supplies are limited it has been decided to vaccinate those most at risk, such as health professionals and pregnant women, and to explain why these persons are more at risk.

> Risks always include some level of uncertainty.... Crisis spokespersons often feel a need to be overly certain and overly reassuring.... However, overly reassuring statements in the face of an inherently uncertain and equivocal situation may reduce a spokesperson's credibility. This is especially the case as a crisis evolves in an unexpected unpredictable way...over reassuring statements that lack credibility may create even higher levels of alarm. (Seeger 2006, p. 241)

6.3.4 All Possible Channels

It is critical that messages come through all possible channels at the same time. A train derailment in Mississauga (a dormitory community just west of Toronto) led to chemicals being released. During the evacuation, Peel Regional police went door to door to make sure everyone in danger was personally warned. But they also broadcast the evacuation decisions over loud hailers so people nearby could hear and they announced them in advance to the media. Everywhere anyone turned they heard the same information. Many heard first from phone calls from persons who had heard the announcement and called to offer assistance (Scanlon and Padgham 1980).

The reason messages must go out on all possible channels at the same time is that people who hear a warning message will check to verify it. If they hear it on the radio they will look to see if it is on TV. They may also ask a family member, friend or neighbour. A study of how persons learned about *two* hurricanes showed that more than 60 % first saw warnings on television, 17–25 % heard first on radio.

If non-media sources come first, then people turn to the media (Kanihan and Gale 2003, p. 89). When the terrorist attacks occurred in the United States on September 11, 2001 and persons were informed by word of mouth, they turned immediately to the mass media, especially television.

> Technically any single communication channel can not meet the information demands.... Our data on citizen preference suggest two important conclusions. First, a mix of channels should be used to send messages. Second, the news media need to be systematically incorporated into this mix. (Perry and Lindell 1989, p. 62)

Although individuals get a great deal of information from the media, they do not necessarily form their opinions from what they hear, read or see. What the media do is make people aware of an issue. But if persons wish to form opinions they consult persons they trust, influencers or opinion leaders, and they consult different persons on different issues (Katz and Lazarsfeld 1955). They might ask a female friend with children about a new infant formula but ask someone they work with about a new union contract. In a health emergency it seems reasonable to suggest they will turn to a physician, a nurse, an ambulance attendant, or even someone with first aid training. If all these people have been given the same information directly they will confirm and therefore support what is being said at news conferences.

6.3.5 *Media Not Homogenous*

Inevitably, there will be rumours. These must be monitored so they can be spotted and stopped. Most research shows rumours stop when they are specifically and clearly denied. Medical professionals should be encouraged to report rumours to officials, as should call centres. Most rumours have some basis in fact.

> When a publicly held view had validity, policy making should be consistent with that view. When a publicly held view is mistaken it should be acknowledged publicly and corrected, not ignored, patronized of ridiculed. (World Health Organization, 2005, p. 6)

There is evidence that media (like officials) tend to think that they must be cautious in reporting frightening information:

> At Three Mile Island, reporters faced a pressure that was new to science reporting. Residents of the area monitored news reports for hints of whether to flee. Overly alarming coverage could have spread panic; overly reassuring coverage could have risked lives. (Stephens and Edison 1982, p. 199)

The same concern showed up after 9/11:

> 'Tom as you point out we try not to exaggerate very much in this circumstance, and yet in many ways it's hard not to exaggerate just the things we have been seeing and the things we are told'—NBC reporter Pat Dawson talking to Tom Brokaw. (Reynolds and Barnett 2003, p. 698)

A study of media coverage of the 1918–1920 influenza pandemic showed that local newspapers tended to downplay the extent of the flu impact in their communities and often ran stories suggesting it was much worse elsewhere (Hurrell et al. 2010). In fact, people find it easier to cope with the truth. It is lack of clarity and confusion that make persons uneasy. It may be necessary to convince health officials and the media of this point. The findings of more than half a century of research into crisis communications have not sunk in.

6.3.6 *Communications Training*

Even a good plan needs to be exercised and those exercises need to include communications. When the New Brunswick Hydro Electric Power Corporation (NBHEPC) ran an emergency exercise for its nuclear power plant, it invited the media. Reporters were invited to ask exactly the questions they would in an emergency. They were welcome to report what was asked and answered if they made clear it was an exercise. The result was that officials faced realistic questions and the public learned how NBHEPC staff would respond. Such practice makes sense:

> Media training should be completed by crisis communicators prior to the onset of a crisis situation. Crises spokespersons should be identified and trained as part of pre-crisis planning. (Seeger 2006, p. 240)

There is always uncertainty during a pandemic and it is important to acknowledge that. It is helpful to explain why a question cannot be answered. In fact, some research suggests experts are more credible when they are less, not more, persuasive. People expect experts to be confident: they apparently pay more attention when they are not (Dehner 2011).

When special operations teams train they assume casualties. A pandemic exercise should do the same: as an exercise is about to start several key players should be told they are not going to participate—and communications personnel should be among them. That is because in a pandemic it is likely that key persons, including designated spokespersons, will become victims. In preparing for a pandemic the exercises should include questions raising ethical concerns. This will force not just spokespersons but those in charge to consider how such issues should be handled.

Because of the increasing use of social media it is now critical to use and monitor outlets such as Twitter and Facebook. During floods in Brisbane, Australia, police used social media to keep the public informed. However, these systems can spread false reports—and those need to be corrected. Given that such systems are not controlled it is more than possible postings will include specific details—who is ill, where they live, etc.—details health authorities may decide not to announce. How should such items be dealt with? A "no comment" is usually taken as a statement the report is accurate; but confirming such reports means the authorities are not in control of communication policy.

Social media do not exist in isolation. They are monitored and used by journalists. Reports on social media will lead to questions from journalists. It is also common for reporters attending a news conference to "tweet" as the conference proceeds. That means it is necessary to provide background before making announcements to avoid the announcement being published out of context. In making corrections, the source must be authoritative: ideally the correction is sent to the person who made the error, allowing him/her to send out the correction.

6.3.7 Early Warning

When a disease outbreak occurs, the most difficult problem may be deciding when there is sufficient evidence to justify a public warning or if a false alarm might lead to the "cry wolf" syndrome—a reluctance to believe future warnings. The latter is a concern at present because it appears the most recent H1N1 outbreak was overblown. There is also the question whether there is a danger of reducing credibility by acting too soon; when tornado warnings are issued, this danger arises if people take shelter and nothing happens for 15 min as people start to think it was a mistake (Simmons and Sutter 2009).

Since a failure to act may lead to charges of a cover-up—who knew what, when?—plus loss of credibility, the consensus is not to delay:

> In today's globalized wired world information about outbreaks is almost impossible to keep hidden from the public. Eventually the outbreak will be revealed. Therefore, to prevent rumours and misinformation . . . it is best to announce as early as possible. . . . (World Health Organization 2005, p. 5)

Despite that consensus, officials sometimes hold back warnings for fear of panic. That can be tragic as shown by what happened when a forest fire threatened a town in Mongolia:

> Officials . . . were convinced that a warning could cause panic: they were reluctant to act unless it was clear there was no other option. They finally broadcast a warning over the radio at 23.00, nearly four hours after the fire struck Xilinji. Most residents were asleep by then. While many got up and moved before the fire struck 10 min later, 25 died. (Xuewen undated)

In fact, people are more likely to ignore warnings than over-react. Yet overcoming the myth of panic may require educating the health community and the media, which has shown the same reluctance because of the same mistaken fear that this could cause alarm or panic.

6.4 Staffing Ethical Issues

A more recent concern during pandemics is the possibility that medical personnel will refuse to work. In 2006, Jacalyn Duffin, professor of History of Medicine at Canada's Queen's University and co-editor of *SARS in Context*, wrote that when an unknown, disease strikes, 'on occasion, doctors and nurses, will sicken, even die, along with their patients.'

> This discouraging lesson pales in contrast to another: medical cowardice will arise. From every valiant doctor who died from the disease being fought, another ran away. (Duffin 2006, p. 3)

A report by the Joint Centre for Bioethics at University of Toronto makes the same claim:

> A significant number of health care workers were infected with SARS because of their work, and some died. Many workers were placed under work quarantine. Workers generally showed heroism and altruism in the face of danger during the SARS outbreak, but some balked at caring for people infected with SARS, and a few were dismissed for failing to report for duty. Post-SARS, many health care workers raised concern about the level of protection to themselves and their families. Some even left their profession. (Pandemic Influenza Working Group 2005, pp. 9–10)

Balicer et al. (2006) and others reported in *BMC Public Health* that roughly half of those surveyed said they would not report to work during a pandemic. Masterson et al. (2009) did a roughly comparable study and found that willingness to report to work dropped when a biological or radioactive agent was involved. Another study reported that approximately one in six public health workers said they would not report to work during a pandemic emergency regardless of its severity. The figures are significantly less than those in a 2005 study conducted by the same research team, in which more than 40 % of public health employees said they were unlikely to report to work during a pandemic. The study also found that workers who thought their jobs were important were more likely to come in (Barnett et al. 2009).

Despite this, it is not clear this will actually happen. People say they may not report in a pandemic but when pandemic strikes they may well do so. Studies of actual behaviour support that conclusion. White (1962) interviewed members of various disaster relief organisations in three communities that had been hit by tornadoes:

> In our random sampling of 128 members of disaster-relief organizations, we found that 77 percent did their jobs first, without serious diversion to family roles. Another five percent were doing rescue work as individuals, so in all 82 percent contributed to disaster relief as the first thing they did. Furthermore, some persons who had first tended to family, or else had done nothing, later came to work. By the end of the first four hours, 89 percent had worked at disaster relief. Not a single person abandoned ongoing disaster work to be with his family. (White 1962)

Russell Dynes and E. L. Quarantelli (1985) found the same thing:

> In sum, in examining a sample of 413 persons who held positions in emergency-relevant organizations, not one abandoned his/her emergency role obligations to opt for familial role obligations.... Consequently ... not a glimmer of support exists for the usual predictions about the consequences of role conflict in emergency situations. The empirical cupboard is so bare that there are no anecdotes to support the conventional wisdom. (Dynes and Quarantelli 1985)

Both those findings were so overwhelming—neither study found a single case of role abandonment—further research seemed pointless. However, these studies focus on fast-onset events. Those involved had to make an immediate decision about what to do. Second, the incidents were over. Those interviewed were not exposed to danger when they responded. It is possible that a pandemic will raise different problems. It builds up over time. It gives people time to ponder. Anyone in contact with victims may believe he or she could become a victim too. Many could think quite rationally that helping someone could be fatal. However, a study in Canada of the 1918–20 Spanish flu showed women volunteered to nurse in hospitals and help in private homes, willingly putting themselves at risk (Scanlon et al. 2009).

However, the possibility that personnel will not show up raises two ethical questions. The first is whether it is ethical for medical personnel to refuse to treat pandemic patients because of the risks. The second is whether to announce such refusals to work, and whether to announce whether any action is being taken against those who refuse. It might seem that reports of such behaviour and disciplinary action would have a deleterious effect on public morale but—given the literature on panic—it would seem preferable to treat the situation transparently. It would be much more damaging for such information to leak or spread through rumours. If the surveys are correct, this could become a serious issue and some thought needs to be given to how it will be handled.

Whether medical personnel respond or not, it is likely a pandemic will lead to a call for volunteers. During the second deadly wave of the so-called Spanish flu in autumn 1918 volunteers were in plentiful supply. Almost all were women and went to work in hospitals or in private homes with a minimum of training (Scanlon et al. 2009). One reason for that response may have been the spirit of volunteerism inspired by war. In addition many of the volunteers were teachers who became available when the schools were closed and in 1918 most teachers were single women. In 1920, more than a year after the war had ended, the Medical Officer of Health in Toronto was reported as saying that volunteers—who had come forward so readily in 1918 when the war was still raging—were not forthcoming:

> Probably the most appalling feature in connection with the present epidemic and one that reflects most upon the people of the so-called 'Christian Toronto' the city of churches, is the fact that in a city of half a million people there cannot be found but a handful that arc willing to come forward and register for volunteer service to their fellow citizens who are in dire need and dire distress. (Twenty-Six Cases Listed By Board 1920)

In 1918 some of those who volunteered had received first aid training as members of the Voluntary Aid Division of St. John Ambulance. Most had attended at the most three or four hours of lectures. Today volunteers would have to be much more carefully briefed and made aware of the risks involved.

6.5 Placarding

In London in the seventeenth century, one regulation required the head of any household to report the presence of plague in his house:

> The Master of every House, as soon as anyone in his House complaineth, either of Botch, or Purple, or swelling in any part of his Body, or falleth otherwise dangerously Sick, without apparent Cause of some other Disease, shall give knowledge thereof to the Examiner of Health, within two hours after the Sign shall appear. (Platt 1997, p. 97–98)

Hodges (1666) reported that once a house was so marked everyone, including neighbours, avoided it. Yet, he says, others could have helped the stricken family. 'I verily believe that many who were lost might have been alive, had not the tragical Mark upon their Doors drove proper Assistances from them (Hodges 1666, p. 9).' He had another criticism:

> ... this Seclusion was ... much the more intolerable, because if a fresh Person was seized in the same House but a Day before another had finished the Quarentine, it was to be performed over again; which occasion'd such tedious Confinements of sick and well together, as sometimes caused the Loss of the whole. (Hodges 1666, p. 7)

Another physician argued some died simply because their spirits sank when they were locked up in a plague-infested house and that made them more likely to get sick:

> It is not easy to conceive a more dismal Scene of Misery than this.... If Fear, Despair, and all Dejection of Spirits dispose the body to receive Contagion and give it a great Power ... as all Physicians agree they do, I don't see how a Disease can be more enforced [spread] than by such a Treatment. (Mead 1720, p. 34)

To make sure everyone remained inside, the residence was locked and watchmen were assigned around the clock to prevent anyone from leaving. That was a virtual death sentence. Shrewsbury called those regulations "barbarous."

However, in 1918–1920, placarding was common in many Ontario communities. Though the provincial government opposed it, municipalities did it anyway. Everyone in such a home was publically tagged a flu victim. No one in the home could work whether or not they had the flu. That was a severe economic penalty. Although placarding was not used during SARS in Toronto some persons were confined to home. Normally one would not expect a person's illnesses to turn them into pariahs the way sex criminals are targeted, yet placarding does just that. However, not to identify high risk individuals may put others unknowingly at risk. This raises the ethical question of whether public concerns must override individual privacy. The University of Toronto Working Group said quarantine was a necessity; but those quarantined needed to be looked after.

> A major flu pandemic could result in very large numbers being subjected to such measures. These restrictions impose a heavy burden on those affected. People may be cut off from family, friends, work, shopping, entertainment, travel and most other activities, including some forms of medical care. People may feel stigmatized.... if quarantine is implemented governments should ensure that people have adequate food supplies and are able to carry out essential functions. Their jobs should be protected and they should not suffer an undue financial burden. (Pandemic Influenza Working Group 2005, p. 13)

Under some conditions privacy rules can be relaxed. For example, if a prison inmate becomes involved in a hostage taking, it is allowable to disclose such information. It may be that during a pandemic privacy rules can be modified in the interests of public safety. Canada's *Privacy Act* for example stipulates that personal information can be disclosed where 'the public interest in disclosure clearly outweighs any invasion of privacy that could result from the disclosure....' (*Privacy Act* R.S.C. 1985 c. P-21 s. 8). The University of Toronto Working Group agreed that was the case in a pandemic:

> The state has a right to override an individual's right to privacy in cases of serious public health risks if revealing private medical information helps to protect public health. (Pandemic Influenza Working Group 2005, p. 13)

This may seem like a legal issue but can it become an ethical one? What if the law is not clear? Are those involved prepared to break the law to inform and protect the public? Will it be necessary to publically justify this decision? The issue becomes more complex if those who are ill are named in the traditional media or on social media as did happen during H1N1: should the authorities confirm the accuracy of these reports?

6.6 Communications About Ethical Issues

Although there is a great deal of discussion about crisis communications, there is little discussion of how ethical issues should be dealt with if they become a matter for public debate. Given the recent research that suggests some medical personnel might decline to show up in a pandemic, it seems reasonable to suggest that if this happens spokespersons for the health authorities are likely to be asked if this behaviour is ethical. They might also be asked what if any steps are being taken to deal with those who fail to show up. Are they being disciplined? Dismissed? If not, why not? It is also possible that someone may ask whether placarding a home, and thus in effect identifying a person who has the flu, is a violation of privacy; or someone could ask whether volunteers are being given access to medical information about the persons they are assisting in hospital or at home.

Some ethical issues would appear to have an obvious and practical answer. The answer to the question of whether an announcement should be made even when there is uncertainty about a disease outbreak seems clear. The announcement should be made and those making it should be both open and restrained, promising further information as it becomes available. To do less risks eventual disclosure that relevant information was concealed. Announcing how a limited amount of vaccine or something like Tamiflu is to be made available is more difficult. Most flu outbreaks hit older people. The 1918–1920 pandemic did not. The problem is that this is likely to become known only after the fact. That means it may be difficult to rationalise some decisions about distribution. There is no question therefore that choices will have to be made. The question is: how far should communicators go in explaining these? Again transparency seems to be the best policy. That means being clear about what data is available and how the decisions reflect that.

In fact, governments have not always been open about such decisions. In autumn 1918 the US Army, with the approval of President Wilson, continued to ship US soldiers overseas even though it was clear many of them would die of the flu en route. The president was admittedly concerned about that policy to the point that he left the White House to pay a personal visit to the US Army Chief of Staff, Peyton March. He acquiesced in the decision when March told him that if such troop shipments were halted it would be a boost to enemy morale (Byerly 2005, p. 5). March is quoted as saying: 'Every such soldier who has died (from influenza) has just as surely played his part as his comrades who have died in France. The shipment of troops should not be stopped for any cause' (Tschanz 2011, p. 1; Iezzoni 1999, p. 104). That decision was not made public and did not become known for more than 80 years. It raises the question as to whether it is ethical for a state to conceal a decision at a time of war.

Other issues are far more complex and would be far more difficult to explain. During past pandemics some persons have died because they were alone, sick and unable to care for themselves. Identifying such persons may require some sort of neighbourhood watch—a request to persons to check on neighbours who live alone. However, as mentioned, this raises special issues during a pandemic. If people do check up on neighbours they may expose themselves to risk. Therefore when this kind of request is issued people need to be told what they should do if they discover someone is ill and what they should do to protect themselves. Of course deciding whether to check on a possibly ill neighbour requires an individual ethical decision. Would it involve an undue risk? Would it make sense, for example, for a parent with three children to expose him or herself to a flu victim? Should a pregnant woman expose herself to such contact?

Far more difficult is the problem of dealing with what is now pervasive privacy legislation. If privacy legislation prohibits certain information from being disclosed then legally it cannot be done. The ethical issue arises when it appears public safety is more important than individual privacy. That means either determining from legal advice that the legislation has an escape clause or it means breaking the law in the interests of public safety. Doing that requires a decision about ethics.

The most difficult ethical issues that may arise in a pandemic are the ones that may occur when the media or others raise ethical issues, for example when—if this happens—medically trained individuals refuse to work and the media or others question whether such behaviour is ethical. While all the existing literature and research suggests transparency is the best policy, none of the literature or research appears to touch on this specific problem. The solution would appear to be—as the literature does suggest—to take a positive approach by finding ways to call attention to the health professionals who are taking the risks because of their commitment. The spokesperson might also point out that other emergency workers such as police and fire-fighters also risk their safety. This might have a second benefit: it would embarrass those who were withholding such services. It might also be wise to have available the relevant code of ethics for professionals. However codes that once stressed that physicians had an obligation to treat patients even if this put their lives in jeopardy no longer state that (Joint Pandemic Working Group undated, p. 11).

One other issue may be whether it is appropriate to announce that some medical personnel are taking advantage of the pandemic to do research, and to spell out the conditions under which people—whether ill or not—will be asked to participate (the focus of Part II of this book). Given the overall evidence that transparency is always the best policy, it would seem appropriate that such research should be made known generally and it should be explained who is doing it, how they are doing it and what people will be told when asked to participate.

6.7 Summary and Conclusions

Although pandemics are rare events, they can be planned for and the kinds of communications issues that will arise can be anticipated. Pandemic planning should identify who will be involved, how they will be kept informed, what sort of issues will likely arise and how they will be dealt with. The planning should identify the various kinds of communication that will have to be done including communication with specific audiences, such as general practitioners and the public. The plans need to review the kinds of questions likely to arise and how they will be answered. The plans should also take into account the fact that there are many ways to get messages out to the public other than the mass media. Most importantly planners should identify spokespersons and their alternates. Given the nature of a pandemic, it is inevitable some key personnel will be among the victims.

There is now enough experience with other types of health emergencies and with other types of emergencies to provide clear guidelines about communications during a pandemic. The best advice is to provide accurate, honest advice, to be as complete as possible and not to conceal any concerns. It is also important not to sound overly professional but to be empathetic and show concern. It is also important to make sure messages are released through all possible channels—including, but not restricted to, the mass media—and that call centres are available for people to contact if they have questions. These centres must be staffed 24/7 and monitored because they are key to finding out what sorts of concerns people have. It is also important there be good lines of communication with physicians, clinics and hospital emergency wards because they, too, need to know what is happening and because they will be continually learning about people's concerns. Communications, in short, is not simply drafting and handing out news releases: it is a carefully planned part of the whole system of crisis response.

Inevitably, as has been made clear, some of these issues will arouse ethical debate. What evidence is necessary for a public warning to be issued or for that warning to be followed by something more serious such as a travel ban? How specific should a community be in issuing pandemic statistics such as the number of confirmed ill or confirmed dead? How should allocation of vaccine be justified? How open should one be in dealing with concerns about the safety of a vaccine? What information about risk must be communicated to volunteers? If, as some believe, some medical personnel will refuse to work during a pandemic how open should officials be about this? How should research initiatives be announced and explained? As should be clear, the best policy is openness and honesty, always put in context. In fact every message about a problem should as far as possible include information about what is being done about that problem.

The main problem in delivering communications related to the threat of or the actual arrival of a pandemic is not in knowing what to do, it is convincing those responsible for communications and the media that transparency is always the best policy. There is significant evidence that officials are reluctant to be open—and for many reasons. While it has been suggested that there are cultural variations in the reasons for this reluctance, and that some do not want to make any statements until there is certainty, the problem is universal.

Disaster research has shown that officials are sometime reluctant to issue warnings for fear of causing panic. In fact panic is so rare it is difficult to study and research suggests that individuals cope best when they are best informed.

References

Balicer, Ran D., Saad B. Omer, Daniel J. Barnett, and George S. Everly. 2006. Local public health workers perceptions' toward responding to an influenza pandemic. *BMC Public Health* 6:99.

Barnett, Daniel J., Ran D. Balicer, Carol B. Thompson, J. Douglas Storey, Saad B. Omer, Natalie L. Semon, Steve Bayer, Lorraine V. Cheek, Kerry W. Gateley, Kathryn M. Lanza, Jane A.

Norbin, Catherine C. Slemp, and Jonathan M. Links. 2009. Assessment of local public health workers' willingness to respond to pandemic influenza through application of the extended parallel process model. *PLoS ONE* 4 (7): e6365.

Byerly, Carol R. 2005. *Fever of war*. New York: New York University Press.

Dehner, George. 2007. Flu: Past and present. *History Compass* 5:709–724.

Duffin, Jacalyn. 2006. Introduction: Lessons and disappointments. In *SARS in context*, eds. Jacalyn Duffin and Arthur Sweetman, 1–15. Kingston: McGill-Queen's University Press.

Dynes, Russell, and Enrico Quarantelli. 1985. *Role simplification in disaster. In Role stressors and support for emergency workers, Center for Mental Health Studies of Emergencies*. Rockville, MD: National Institute of Mental Health.

Hodges, Nathaniel. 1666. Loimologia.

Iezzoni, Lynette. 1999. Influenza, 1918: The worst epidemic in American history. TV Books.

Joint Pandemic Working Group. n.d. Ethics and SARS: Learning lessons from the Toronto experience. Toronto: Joint Centre for Bioethics.

Kanihan, Stacey Frank, and Kendra L. Gale. 2003. Within 3 hours, 97 percent learn about 9/11 attacks. *Media Studies of September 11* 24:78–92.

Katz, Elihu, and Paul F. Lazarsfeld. 1955. *Personal influence*. Glencoe, IL: The Free Press.

Kraul, M. 2010. Immigration, ethnicity and the pandemic. *Public Health Reports* 125 (Suppl 3): 123–133.

Masterson, Lori, Christel Steffen, Michael Brin, Mary Frances Kordick, and Steve Christos. 2009. Willingness to respond of emergency department personnel and their predicted participation in mass casualty terrorist events. *Journal of Emergency Medicine* 36 (1): 43–49.

Mead, Richard. 1720. *A short discourse concerning pestilential contagion and the methods used to prevent it*. London: S. Buckley.

Pandemic Influenza Working Group. 2005. *Stand on guard for thee*. Toronto: Joint Centre for Bioethics.

Perry, Ron, and Michael Lindell. 1989. *Communicating environmental risk in multiethnic communities*. London: Sage.

Platt, Colin. 1997. *King Death: The Black Death and its aftermath in late-medieval England*. Toronto: University of Toronto Press.

Privacy, Act, Revised Statutes of Canada 1985, c. P-21, s. 8.

Reynolds, Amy, and Brooke Barnett. 2003. This just in . . . How national TV news handled the breaking 'live' coverage of September 11. *Journalism & Mass Communication Quarterly* 80:689–703.

Scanlon, Joseph, with Massey Padgham. 1980. *The Peel Regional Police Force & The Mississauga Evacuation*. Ottawa: Canadian Police College.

Scanlon, Joseph, Terry McMahon, and Casey Hurrell. 2009. Almost only women: Canadian volunteer response to the 1918–20 pandemic. *American Journal of Disaster Medicine* 4:331–344.

Seeger, Matthew W. 2006. Best practices in crisis communication: An expert panel process. *Journal of Applied Communication Research* 34:232–244.

Simmons, Kevin, and Dan Sutter. 2009. False alarms, tornado warnings and tornado casualties. *Weather, Climate and Society* 1:38–53.

Sims, Hugh Joffre. 1984. *Sims' history of Elgin County*. Shedden: Elgin County Library.

Stephens, Mitchell, and Nadyne Edison. 1982. An analysis of news media coverage of issues at Three Mile Island. *Journalism Quarterly* 59:199–204.

Tschanz, David W. 2011. Plague of the Spanish Lady. Military History Online. http://www.militaryhistoryonline.com/wwi/articles/plagueofspanishlady.aspx. Accessed 1 May 2013.

Twenty-Six cases listed by board. 1920. The Morning Chronicle, February 14, p. 4.

White, Meda Miller. 1962. *Role conflict in disasters: Not family but familiarity first*. Chicago: University of Chicago.

World Health Organization. 2005. *WHO outbreak communication guidelines*. Geneva: World Health Organization.

Xuewen, Sheng. n.d. Emergency response in the People's Republic of China: A case study of the 1987 Daxinganling forest fire. Unpublished paper.

Chapter 7
Evidence and Healthcare Needs During Disasters

Aasim Ahmad, Syed Mamun Mahmud and Dónal P. O'Mathúna

7.1 Introduction

Disasters cause much damage and inflict much human suffering. They lead to severe imbalances between human needs and the resources immediately available to meet those needs (Wang 2009). Disasters come in many different types. The Centre for Research on the Epidemiology of Disasters (CRED) maintains a publicly accessible database called the Emergency Events Database (EM-DAT). This categorises disasters into one of three groups: natural disasters (e.g. floods, earthquakes, mudslides), technological disasters (e.g. industrial accidents, transport accidents), or combinations of these in what are called complex emergencies (CRED 2011). Disasters can also be conflict-related (due to, for example, war or terrorism), and these may or may not be considered separately.

The lack of standard definitions has led to much variability in the data available on disasters in different databases (Kar-Purkayasha et al. 2011). This leads to varying estimates of the precise impacts and costs of disasters. Such databases are the result of considerable effort and resources, and they contain large amounts of data. Even with their limitations, such databases provide a general sense of the disaster trends. According to CRED, the number of natural disasters is increasing steadily, with 2010 being the deadliest year in decades: 373 natural disasters killed almost 300,000 people, impacted over 200 million more, and cost over US$100 billion (CRED 2011). Foremost amongst these, the Haiti earthquake killed over 222,000 people and a heat wave in Russia killed about 56,000 people; the costliest disaster in 2010 was an earthquake in Chile estimated to have caused US$30 billion in damages.

A. Ahmad (✉)
Aga Khan University, Karachi, Pakistan
e-mail: aasimahmad@gmail.com

S. M. Mahmud
The Kidney Centre Post Graduate Training Institute, Karachi, Pakistan

D. P. O'Mathúna
Dublin City University, Dublin, Ireland

D. P. O'Mathúna et al. (eds.), *Disaster Bioethics: Normative Issues When Nothing is Normal,* Public Health Ethics Analysis 2, DOI 10.1007/978-94-007-3864-5_7,

At the same time, some positive developments are occurring. According to the *2011 Global Assessment Report on Disaster Risk Reduction*, the risk of death due to weather-related disasters is decreasing globally, except for those who live in the poorest countries (United Nations 2011). However, the economic cost of disasters is increasing in all parts of the world. The forecast does not look good. One assessment found that climate-related disasters (which make up 98 % of all disasters) will affect about 375 million people annually by 2015, an increase of 50 % over recent averages (Ganeshan and Diamond 2009). The financial loss from Japan's 2011 earthquake and tsunami alone was estimated at more than US$300 billion (CNN 2011).

As the frequency of natural disasters increases, their impact is especially significant in lower income countries. Ironically, as countries begin to experience economic growth, their exposure to economic loss from disasters increases more rapidly (United Nations 2011). Underlying factors that contribute to these additional risks are poverty, bad urban planning and management, and ecosystem decline. The impact of a disaster on ecology, health, and economics largely depends on the type of disaster and the underlying characteristics of the community, the geo-political state of the region, and the population's vulnerability and capacity to respond. New evidence is showing that disasters have a particularly negative impact on children and displaced persons, yet these are rarely taken into account (United Nations 2011).

Despite the growing knowledge about disaster prevention and disaster risk reduction, dealing with disasters and their aftermath has always been difficult, even in regions with financially sound and well established systems, as was seen with Hurricane Katrina. This is because the nature and magnitude of disasters is highly variable and the conditions and needs are usually not known accurately in the immediate aftermath of a disaster.

Disasters result in what have been called the 6 Ds: destruction, death, disease/disorders, displacement, disappearance, and disarray (Sumathipala et al. 2010). Most of these have implications for the healthcare needs of those affected by disasters. Responses to those needs, like all healthcare decisions, should be based on high-quality rigorous research and evidence. Unfortunately, current decision-makers in disaster situations are often without the high quality research and sound evidence they would like to have. More generally, 'much of the existing operational research related to emergencies and disasters lacks consistency, is of poor reliability and validity and is of limited use for establishing baselines, defining standards, making comparisons or tracking trends' (UNISDR 2011, p. 46). All this points to the importance of generating evidence to guide healthcare workers and policy-makers. This leads to questions concerning what evidence is needed, how it should be generated and the ethical issues involved in conducting research to produce such evidence.

7.2 Evidence-based Practice

Evidence can be defined as various observations, facts or organised bodies of information offered to support or justify inferences or beliefs provided to support various conclusions or judgements (Bradt 2009a). Evidence-based medicine (EBM) has developed since the early 1990s in response to concerns about the way clinical decisions were made prior to then. EBM is defined as 'The conscientious, explicit, and judicious use of current best evidence in making decisions about the care of individual patients. The practice of evidence-based medicine requires the integration of individual clinical expertise with the best available external clinical evidence from systematic research and our patient's unique values and circumstances' (Bradt 2009a, p. 299). Prior to this, it had been assumed that informed intuition, unsystematic observations from clinical experience, pathophysiological rationale, and traditional medical training were sufficient for clinical decision-making (Bradt 2009a). In what has been described as a Kuhnian 'paradigm shift', EBM developed, stressing the examination of evidence from clinical research (Kuhn 1970).

Given the heterogeneity of modern health care systems, it is naïve to expect a univocal definition of evidence. Although EBM arose from clinical epidemiology, a quantitative discipline, quantitative approaches alone will not be sufficient to assess the strength of all forms of evidence relevant to EBM. Critics of EBM describe it as representative of narrow reductionism that inappropriately relies on epidemiology and statistics, while ignoring clinical judgment and experience. Evidence within EBM is ranked hierarchically, with highest place given to systematic reviews and randomised controlled trials (Bradt 2009a). While qualitative methods either are not included in such hierarchies or are given lower priority, this arises because of the types of questions addressed by each research methodology. EBM focuses on questions of effectiveness and safety of interventions, for which a randomised controlled trial (RCT) is best suited.

Such an approach does not mean that qualitative methodologies are not appreciated to address other questions. At the very least, values, preferences and experiences of individuals and communities must be incorporated into clinical decision-making. It is certainly not enough to have quantitative evidence alone to measure the strength of evidence, but individual preferences and contextual dimensions must be taken into account. Attention to the narrative context of clinical care explains the extent to which values and experiences are seen as relevant evidence, but more importantly underscores the significance of how evidence is collected and interpreted (Greenhalgh 1997). Thus, it is not that EBM per se is problematic, but rather that the importance of carefully choosing one's clinical question may be overlooked. This then impacts how decisions are made about what type of evidence is most applicable and needed.

The changes promoted by EBM have taken decades to materialise. The role of evidence-based practice in humanitarian relief of disasters is only now being developed, and faces a number of challenges. Within EBM, external evidence takes higher priority over expert opinion, yet within disaster relief settings, expert opinion continues to reign supreme (Bradt 2009b). Within disaster relief, local and context-specific knowledge remains important but needs to be combined with 'global' evidence (Kayabu and Clarke 2013).

Humanitarian responses should be based on needs, and evidence plays an important role in identifying needs accurately and showing how needs can best be met, especially with limited resources. But the acute crisis of a disaster can leave needs assessment and evidence accumulation as lower priorities. 'Without appropriate evidence, allocation is based on estimates and professional judgement, and needs assessments in practice play a minor part in determining allocations' (Willitts-King 2006, p. 26). A vicious cycle can be set up where the lack of evidence makes evidence-based decisions impossible, leading to a lack of incentives to develop the needed evidence.

7.2.1 Evidence-based Guidelines

When evidence is lacking in any healthcare arena, decision-making guidelines tend to be less helpful. For example, analysis of various medical guidelines has found that developers use a puzzling variety of systems to rate the quality of evidence underlying their recommendations. 'Some are facile, some confused, and others sophisticated but complex' (Guyatt et al. 2008b, p. 995).

To address this situation and improve clinical decision-making, formal systems have been developed to grade the quality of evidence available and the strength of recommendation possible. While these have been developed primarily to assist in normal medical situations, these can be usefully applied in disaster settings. A variety of systems and tools have been developed, with the GRADE approach (Grading of Recommendations Assessment, Development and Evaluation) being one which is increasingly being adopted by organisations worldwide (Guyatt et al. 2008a). The GRADE system is explicit, comprehensive, transparent and pragmatic in its approach. It has similarities to other grading systems, but seeks to incorporate all of the advantages available in other systems. It is beyond the scope of this chapter to examine the GRADE approach extensively, but some of its key factors will be mentioned.

Central to the GRADE approach is making a distinction between rating the quality of evidence and grading the strength of recommendations (Guyatt et al. 2008a). Quality of evidence refers to the types of studies conducted to address a research question and relates to the level of confidence we can have in the current estimate of effect. For example, in addressing whether or not an intervention is effective, RCTs provide the highest quality evidence and anecdotal reports provide low quality evidence, also called a high risk of bias.

Strength of recommendation differs significantly from the quality of evidence, although the terms are sometimes used interchangeably. If the two are not clearly distinguished, confusion can result (Guyatt et al. 2008a). A strong recommendation may be given if high quality evidence consistently supports a particular intervention. Sometimes lower quality evidence (say, observational studies) can support a strong recommendation if the beneficial effect is consistently large and adverse effects minimal. At the same time, high quality evidence may lead to a weak recommendation if, for example, the desirable and undesirable effects are relatively balanced, or if the evidence shows that different interventions are similarly effective (Jaeschke et al. 2008). In such cases, even if high quality evidence exists, choosing whether or not to use an intervention, or picking between interventions, will need to rely more on cultural or individual values.

Another factor is how well a specific research study has been designed and conducted. While RCTs will normally be high-quality evidence, their quality can be reduced by study design limitations (lack of blinding, subjective outcomes, etc.), inconsistent results across different studies, indirectness of evidence, imprecision (primarily due to small sample sizes) or publication bias (Guyatt et al. 2008b). Lower quality studies may have their quality increased if large magnitude effects are consistently found, if all plausible biases would reduce the demonstrated effect, or if a dose-response gradient is visible (Guyatt et al. 2008b).

Because of the importance of using evidence to guide disaster responses, many organisations are recognising the need to evaluate guidelines along the lines of those suggested by GRADE. For example, the World Bank has described four general models of research methodology for conducting impact evaluation of interventions in humanitarian settings (World Bank undated; Independent Evaluation Group 2009).

1. Randomised evaluation. Groups or locations are randomly assigned to receive different interventions or controls. Outcome measures are collected or other observations gathered to assess the impact of the interventions.
2. Quasi-experimental design where the intervention group is matched to a control group by non-random methods. Statistical methods are used to ensure the groups are as similar as possible.
3. Ex-post comparison of intervention group with a non-equivalent control group. Evaluation occurs after the project has started and multivariate analysis is used to control for differences between the groups.
4. Non-experimental approaches using surveys and case studies to collect information on perceptions of interventions' impact.

The World Bank regards only Types 1 and 2 as rigorous because 'they are the most reliable for establishing causality—the relationship between a specific intervention and actual impacts—and for estimating the magnitude of impact attributable to the intervention. They are able to distinguish the impacts of the intervention from the influence of other, external factors' or confounders (World Bank undated, p. 3). While these methods are the most reliable for certain questions, the World Bank also notes that qualitative studies remain valuable, with mixed method approaches having many advantages.

7.3 Evidence and Disasters

Having discussed the complex issues of evidence and evidence-based approaches in general, the role of evidence for decision-making in disaster settings will be examined more closely. Currently most disaster relief operations are based on evidence that not too infrequently is of questionable accuracy and low quality. Although rigorous approaches to evaluation are necessary to provide the best guidance during disasters, 'the limited corpus of rigorous studies is notable' (Bradt 2009b, p. 488). As a result, decision-making in disaster management is largely dependent on expert opinion, eminence-based decisions or non-rigorous studies (Bradt 2009b).

In such situations, well-meaning healthcare professionals do the best they can, but can make decisions that do not have good outcomes. The first author of this chapter witnessed this after a recent earthquake in Pakistan.

> A 4 year old girl child was brought to the children's hospital in Islamabad 3 weeks after the devastating earthquake that hit the northern areas of Pakistan in early October 2005. She had an amputated right arm, with disarticulated elbow joint and a jutting humerus, without any muscle cover. It so transpired that the initial surgery was performed in a makeshift camp by the surgeons of an international aid organization. Not one of the doctors involved was a qualified surgeon. (Loff et al. 2007, p. 265)

To avoid such well-intentioned, but non-evidence based decision-making, other surgical teams undertook research after the same earthquake to provide evidence that could be applied to future disaster relief efforts after earthquakes (Rajpura et al. 2010). By involving international and local medical expertise, evidence about how best to treat complex fractures was developed to save as many limbs as possible while promoting optimal patient care.

Little is documented during disaster relief, which hinders learning from past experience. When data is collected, it is usually not standardised, leading to much variability in the available databases. Research reports have contained insufficient detail, revealed shortcomings in study methodology, and raised concerns about high risk of bias. All this, in spite of 'an ethical imperative to ensure that all data collected is of good quality, and is useful and relevant to as many users as possible' (Kar-Purkayasha et al. 2011, p. 10). The resulting challenges are being tackled by a number of initiatives, including the Cochrane Collaboration's Evidence Aid, the US National Library of Medicine's Disaster Information Management Research Center, the World Association for Disaster and Emergency Medicine (WADEM) and the UK Wellcome Trust.

Systematic reviews of randomised double-blind placebo-controlled studies provide the highest quality evidence for interventions and can lead to the strongest recommendations, but these are practically non-existent for disaster situations—and sometimes ethically impossible to conduct. However, they are widely recognised as crucial to developing evidence-based disaster response (Kayabu and Clarke 2013). When available, they can contribute to developing globally accepted standards for performance and accountability during disaster relief operations. In addition, while accreditation standards for those responding to disasters are not generally available, a register for disaster healthcare professionals was recently established in the UK (Redmond 2011).

7.4 Evidence and Ethics in Disasters

The underlying motivations for generating and using evidence in disaster settings is ethical. The primary objective in disaster relief, as in all humanitarian assistance, is to do the most good for as many people as possible (Bradt 2009b). In the immediate aftermath of a disaster, this involves saving lives and alleviating suffering. However, myths and fallacies about health risks and health needs during disasters exist in both public perceptions and the views of some responders (Wang 2009). Good quality evidence is needed to identify the best ways to help people after disasters.

For example, panic is believed to be widespread after a disaster, yet evidence shows that most survivors do not panic. Instead, empirical research has for long shown that survivors remain calm and play crucial roles as the first responders to help rescue people and treat their injuries (Quarantelli 1975). Although external disaster response teams play important roles, empirical research in China, Mexico and the US has found that more than 80 % of disaster survivors are located and rescued by other survivors (Wang 2009). This has important implications for disaster preparedness training and planning, highlighting the importance of conducting research immediately after disasters.

For example, to address the trauma associated with disasters, different psychological interventions have been used widely. Rather than assuming that any intervention by a caring, competent counsellor is helpful, research is identifying which interventions are effective and for which people. A systematic review of research on psychological debriefing to prevent post-traumatic stress disorder (PTSD) has shown that it is generally not effective (Rose et al. 2002). On the other hand, for those exhibiting PTSD symptoms, cognitive behavioural therapy (CBT) can be safe and effective (Kar 2011). However, up to 50 % of those treated do not respond to CBT for a variety of reasons.

Another important ethical principle is to avoid harm. Disaster responses must be examined with a long-term perspective, not just short-term. Thus, an evaluation of the response to the 2004 Indian Ocean Tsunami has found that the influx of foreign aid undermined local disaster relief efforts and, in places, set back local organisational infrastructural (Cosgrave 2007). Such outcomes were surely unintended, but 'good intentions do not excuse bad outcomes' (Bradt 2009b, p. 483). High quality evidence can help identify why these harms resulted and how they can be avoided with different interventions. Another finding is that local communities did much to save lives in the immediate aftermath of the Tsunami. This highlights the importance of investing in disaster risk reduction and preparedness as an effective means of reducing future harms (Cosgrave 2007). The importance of local communities has often been overlooked, but now there is good quality evidence to support their importance.

One of the central ethical principles of humanitarian assistance is that resources should be provided according to need (Willitts-King 2006). One of the reasons for this approach is to minimise the provision of resources according to bias or prejudice, such as when one group receives more or less aid because of race, religion, gender, age, social class or other non-relevant attribute. If aid is not provided according to need, further harm can occur to those with the greater needs who do not receive sufficient aid. In addition, needs-based assistance is a just way of distributing scare resources.

Providing aid according to need necessitates prior understanding of people's needs. However, accurate data on people's needs is often limited, especially in the immediate aftermath of disasters. A number of international humanitarian initiatives have found serious deficits in the information available on health needs requiring humanitarian assistance and a lack of standardised approaches to collecting such data (Bradt 2009b).

Conducting needs assessments in disaster settings is challenging, and points to the importance of awareness of pre-disaster health resources and infrastructure. Once again, the overall value of the evidence from needs assessments provides some ethical justification for carrying out such studies. At the same time, many ethical challenges exist for such research in disaster settings. Collecting accurate data is pivotal, but difficult during a disaster. A balance must be maintained between the immediate needs of individuals and the long-term needs of the population at large.

While evidence is both vital and scarce in disaster relief settings, evidence and knowledge are not the main limiting factors to effective humanitarian responses. 'Rather, it was (the lack) of political and organizational will to act on that knowledge, and to deploy the necessary resources to tackle problems using the best available solutions' (Bradt 2009b, p. 482). Such issues go to the underlying moral motivations of those involved in disaster relief, which go beyond the focus of this chapter.

7.5 Ethical Challenges in Disaster Research

Evidence-based practice, as shown by the examples given above, demonstrates the need for, and value of, disaster research. However, how such research is conducted raises a number of different ethical issues. A number of these will be addressed in depth in Part II of this book, so they will be mentioned only briefly here. Such ethical issues in disaster research range from the difficulty in assessing benefits and risks (Chap. 8), the quality or lack thereof of truly 'informed' consent (Chap. 9), the vulnerability of participants (Chap. 11), appropriate standards of care, and the 'philanthropic' misconception, to the paucity of ethical guidelines for disaster situations and the difficulties for members of research ethics committees to review complicated protocols urgently and thoroughly (Chap. 12).

7.5.1 Ethical Guidelines

Ethical guidelines for research (both national and international) can contribute to the appropriate conduct of research in disaster situations. However, specific guidelines for disaster research are lacking. One such set of guidelines was developed by the Working Group on Disaster Research and Ethics (WGDRE) which was formed in response to the 2004 Indian Ocean tsunami (Sumathipala et al. 2010). These guidelines are intended to supplement, not replace, existing research ethics guidelines by highlighting ethical issues of particular importance in disaster settings. They articulate twelve general principles, which are briefly summarised below.

1. All research in disaster situations should be relevant to those affected by disasters and impossible to conduct in non-disaster situations.
2. Informed consent for research is mandatory. While prior, free and voluntary informed consent is difficult to attain in normal circumstances, it is particularly challenging in disaster situations. Informed consent for medical or scientific

research is a 'non-derogable right' and therefore cannot be exempted if individuals have the capacity (UN Commission on Human Rights 1984). Research teams should identify potential barriers to informed consent and make every effort to overcome them. Inducement of any kind must be avoided and no attempt made to disguise research as humanitarian aid or part thereof. Efforts must be made to avoid the so-called 'philanthropic misconception' (Ahmad and Mahmud 2010). This is a specific instance of the therapeutic misconception where research subjects believe their participation in a study is equivalent to clinical care and confuse the researcher with a care giver. Disaster victims may similarly confuse research participation with humanitarian aid.

3. Community consultation and participation should be encouraged at all stages of the research process. At the same time, collective community agreements should not substitute for individual informed consent.
4. Research participants should be selected for scientific reasons related to the research project. The research should not put extra burdens on those who are already traumatized or the local infrastructure.
5. Extra care should be taken to protect the privacy, confidentiality and dignity of survivors.
6. While disaster survivors may not be defined legally as a vulnerable population (Levine 2004), their heightened vulnerability should lead to additional efforts to minimise risks from the research.
7. Institutions sponsoring disaster research should recognise their ethical obligations and help coordinate research with disaster relief.
8. The highest standards of professional competence and scientific rigour should be maintained within the research team.
9. The research should provide direct or indirect benefits to those researched, the disaster-affected community or future disaster victims. The local community should be consulted regarded those benefits.
10. The research results should be disseminated widely and transparently after peer-review, and used to influence policy.
11. Independent, multidisciplinary and pluralist ethics committees should review all research proposals. Representatives from the disaster-affected community should be included. Novel arrangements and different stages of review may need to be developed.
12. International collaborative research must be based on mutual respect and partnership, involving various organisations and the local community.

7.6 Conclusion

Much further work needs to be done on generating evidence for disaster situations, working to ensure decisions made in disaster planning and responses are evidence-based, and ensuring that research is conducted to the highest ethical standards. The

WGDRE guidelines provide an important foundation for the development of international guidelines for disaster research (Sumathipala et al. 2010). Standards of care in disaster situations have been defined in different ways, making it challenging to see to what standards healthcare providers and researchers should be held accountable (Altevogt et al. 2009; Annas 2010). Given this lack of clarity, review by a research ethics committee is particularly important. However, ethical review of disaster research is challenging given the urgency of review, the devastation and complexity in the research setting, and the importance of training all committee members. Some frameworks for ethics committees have been proposed, but further work is needed in this area (Schopper et al. 2009; Tansey et al. 2011). Disaster bioethics is a complex and multi-faceted field of study, with much challenging analysis and discussion remaining to be done.

References

Ahmad, Aasim, and Syed Maum Mahmud. 2010. Philanthropic misconception. *Asian Bioethics Review* 2: 154–161.

Altevogt, Bruce M., Clare Stroud, Sarah L. Hanson, Dan Hanfling, and Lawrence O. Gostin, eds. 2009. Guidance for establishing crisis standards of care for use in disaster situations: A letter report. Washington, DC: National Academies Press.

Annas, George J. 2010. Standard of care—In sickness and in health and in emergencies. *New England Journal of Medicine* 362: 2126–2131.

Bradt, David A. 2009a. Evidence-based decision-making (part 1): Origins and evolution in the health sciences. *Prehospital and Disaster Medicine* 24: 298–305.

Bradt, David A. 2009b. Evidence-based decision-making (part 2): Applications in disaster relief operations. *Prehospital and Disaster Medicine* 24: 479–492.

CNN. 2011. Official: Quake, tsunami could cost Japan $300 billion. CNN World. http://articles.cnn.com/2011-03-31/world/japan.disaster.budget_1_tsunami-quake-yen?_s=PM:WORLD. Accessed 2 February 2012.

Cosgrave, John. 2007. Synthesis report: Expanded summary. Joint evaluation of the international response to the Indian Ocean tsunami. London: Tsunami Evaluation Coalition. http://www.alnap.org/pool/files/Syn_Report_Sum.pdf. Accessed 2 February 2012.

CRED. 2011. Killer year caps deadly decade—reducing disaster impact is "critical" says top UN disaster official. http://www.unisdr.org/archive/17613. Accessed 2 February 2012.

Ganeshan, Shamanthy, and Wayne Diamond. 2009. Forecasting the numbers of people affected annually by natural disasters up to 2015. Oxfam GB. http://www.oxfam.org/sites/www.oxfam.org/files/forecasting-disasters-2015.pdf. Accessed 2 February 2012.

Greenhalgh, Trisha. 1997. From EBM to CSM: The evolution of context-sensitive medicine. *Journal of Evaluation in Clinical Practice* 3: 105–108.

Guyatt, Gordon H., Andrew D. Oxman, Gunn E. Vist, Regina Kunz, Yngve Falck-Ytter, Pablo Alonso-Coello, and Holger J. Schünemann, for the GRADE Working Group. 2008a. GRADE: An emerging consensus on rating quality of evidence and strength of recommendations. *British Medical Journal* 336: 924–926.

Guyatt, Gordon H., Andrew D. Oxman, Gunn E. Vist, Regina Kunz, Yngve Falck-Ytter, Pablo Alonso-Coello, and Holger J. Schünemann, for the GRADE Working Group. 2008b. GRADE: What is "quality of evidence" and why is it important to clinicians? *British Medical Journal* 336: 995–998.

Independent, Evaluation Group. 2009. Institutionalizing impact evaluation within the framework of a monitoring and evaluation system. Washington, DC: World Bank. http://siteresources.worldbank.org/EXTEVACAPDEV/Resources/4585672-1251461875432/inst_ie_framework_me.pdf. Accessed 2 February 2012.

Jaeschke, Roman., Gordon H. Guyatt, Phil Dellinger, Holger Schünemann, Mitchell M Levy, Regina Kunz, Susan Norris, Julian Bion, for the GRADE working group. 2008. Use of GRADE grid to reach decisions on clinical practice guidelines when consensus is elusive. *British Medical Journal* 337: 327–330.

Kar, N. 2011. Cognitive behavioral therapy for the treatment of post-traumatic stress disorder: A review. *Neuropsychiatric Disease and Treatment* 7:167–181.

Kar-Purkayasha, Ishani., Mike Clarke, and Virginia Murray. 2011. Dealing with disaster databases—What can we learn from health and systematic reviews? PLOS Currents Disasters (last modified: 2012 Aug 29). Edition 1. doi:10.1371/currents.RRN1272.

Kayabu, Bonnix., and Mike Clarke. 2013. The use of systematic reviews and other research evidence in disasters and related areas: Preliminary report of a needs assessment survey. PLOS Currents Disasters. (Last modified: 2013 Jan 22). Edition 1. doi:10.1371/currents.dis.ed42382881b3bf79478ad503be4693ea.

Kuhn, Thomas S. 1970. *The structure of scientific revolutions*. Chicago: University of Chicago Press.

Levine, Carol. 2004. The concept of vulnerability in disaster research. *Journal of Traumatic Stress* 17: 395–402.

Loff, Bebe., Brad Crammond, Robyna Khan, Aasim Ahmad, and Deborah Zion. 2007. *Ethical considerations in humanitarian and development aid: What have we learnt over the last 20 years? In Measuring effectiveness in humanitarian and development aid: Conceptual frameworks, principles and practice*, ed. André M. N. Renzaho, 259–277. New York: Nova Science.

Quarantelli, Enrico L. 1975. Panic behavior: Some empirical observations. Disaster Research Center. http://dspace.udel.edu:8080/dspace/bitstream/handle/19716/393/PP20.pdf?sequence=3. Accessed 2 February 2012.

Rajpura, Asim., Ihab Boutros, Tahir Khan, and Sohail A. Khan. 2010. Pakistan earthquake: Experiences of a multidisciplinary surgical team. *Prehospital and Disaster Medicine* 25: 361–367.

Redmond, Anthony D., Timothy J. O'Dempsey, and Bertrand Taithe. 2011. Disasters and a register for foreign medical teams. *Lancet* 377: 1054–1055.

Rose, S. C., J. Bisson, R. Churchill, and S. Wessely. 2002. Psychological debriefing for preventing post traumatic stress disorder (PTSD). Cochrane Database of Systematic Reviews Issue 2.

Schopper, Doris., Ross Upshur, Francine Matthys, Jerome A. Singh, Sunita S. Bandewar, Aasim Ahmad, and Els van Dongen. 2009. Research ethics review in humanitarian contexts: The experience of the Ethics Review Board of Médecins Sans Frontières. *PLoS Medicine* 6: e1000115.

Sumathipala, Athula., Amir Jafarey, Leonardo D. de Castro, Aasim Ahmad, Darryl Marcer, Sandya Srinivasan, Nandini Kumar, Sisira Siribaddana, Sleman Sutaryo, Anant Bhan, Dananjaya Waidyaratne, Sriyakanthi Beneragama, Chandrani Jayasekera, Sarath Edirisingha, and Chesmal Siriwardhana. 2010. Ethical issues in post-disaster clinical interventions and research: A developing world perspective. Key findings from a drafting and consensus generation meeting of the Working Group on Disaster Research and Ethics (WGDRE) 2007. *Asian Bioethics Review* 2: 124–142.

Tansey, Catherine M., Margaret S. Herridge, Ronald J. Heslegrave, and James V. Lavery. 2011. A framework for ethics review during public emergencies. *Canadian Medical Association Journal* 182: 1533–1537.

UNISDR. 2011. Hyogo Framework for Action 2005–2015. Building the resilience of nations and communities to disasters. Mid-term review 2010–2011. http://www.unisdr.org/we/inform/publications/1037. Accessed 2 February 2012.

United Nations. 2011. Global assessment report on disaster risk reduction. http://www.unisdr.org/we/inform/publications/19846.

United Nations Commission on Human Rights. 1984. The Siracusa principles on the limitation and derogation provisions in the international covenant on civil and political rights. http://www.unhcr.org/refworld/docid/4672bc122.html. Accessed 2 February 2012.

Wang, Tzong-Luen. 2009. Common myths and fallacies in disaster medicine: An evidence-based review. *Fu-Jen Journal of Medicine* 7: 149–160.

Willitts-King, Barnaby. Practical approaches to needs-based allocation of humanitarian aid: A review for Irish Aid on donor approaches. http://reliefweb.int/node/22572. Accessed 2 February 2012.

World Bank. undated. OED and impact evaluation—A discussion note. http://www.worldbank.org/oed/docs/world_bank_oed_impact_evaluations.pdf. Accessed 2 February 2012.

Part II
Research Ethics and Disasters

Chapter 8
Interests Divided: Risks to Disaster Research Subjects vs. Benefits to Future Disaster Victims

Evelyne Shuster

8.1 Introduction

In this chapter I will argue, along with Paul Farmer, that for disaster victims 'research [on humans] is always a luxury' (Farmer 2005, p. 205). This conclusion is reachable by many routes, and I will concentrate on conducting an ethical harm-benefit analysis that treats victims of disasters as persons who are ends in themselves and who cannot be placed at excessive risk, only for the benefits of others. 'Research' is a 'systematic investigation ... designed to develop or contribute to generalizable knowledge' (US Code of Federal Regulations 1976). Of course, there are different kinds of research. Not all research *involving* human beings is research *on* human beings, nor is there a "*one size fits all*" rule that applies to all types of disasters. Considerations in war are different from those in flood, earthquake, or famine. And the research method matters. Epidemiological research, including surveillance data collection and monitoring strategies to guide fair and efficient allocation of limited resources, for example, are reasonable and may even be required in the immediate aftermath of radiation exposure or in an epidemic outbreak of a viral disease (Barzilay 2013). The Presidential Commission for the Study of Bioethical Issues has provided the ethical framework for the conduct of emergency research on pre- and post-event of [anthrax vaccine adsorbed post exposure prophylaxis] in children (Presidential Commission 2013). But biomedical (or clinical) research that involves physical, psychological or dignitary harm to research subjects is difficult to justify in the immediate response to a disaster—although it may be ethically acceptable during the next phase, i.e., the recovery phase of a disaster.

Disasters can claim more or fewer victims based on the magnitude of the damages they cause and the immediate response of humanitarian workers. First responders can be acclaimed as heroic rescuers one moment, and later denounced as self-interested looters. Researchers are not immune: they may be acclaimed as helpful scientists who

E. Shuster (✉)
Veterans Affairs Medical Center,
Philadelphia, USA
e-mail: evelyn1@seas.upenn.edu

D. P. O'Mathúna et al. (eds.), *Disaster Bioethics: Normative Issues When Nothing is Normal*, Public Health Ethics Analysis 2, DOI 10.1007/978-94-007-3864-5_8,

produce new knowledge for the benefit of society at one moment, and then denounced as exploiters of human tragedy for their personal interests. Researchers may think that 'without testing the outcomes of a potential new therapy in an actual emergency situation, it is impossible to improve practices in order to limit the damage in future situations. Research is necessary' (Reed 2002, p. 10). Researchers may even view 'war as an amazing learning environment, the perfect laboratory for ... research ... [and argue that war] injuries are too rare to study in peacetime. [And thus] continuous research is not only desirable ... [it] ought to be ... obligatory' (Bohannon 2011, pp. 1261–1263). The goals of *research* and *rescue* may seem compatible and obligatory, just as the integration of *research* and *care* has appeared ethically necessary (Largent et al. 2011). Harvard professor Jennifer Leaning aptly asked:

> Are ... clinical studies (such as severe malnutrition in children and adults) in which the unavoidable trade-off in risk and benefit is accentuated by the irreducible uncertainty of achieving truly informed and unforced consent, ever justifiable? The [research] field response is yes. Work with populations whose lives are at grave risk and dependent upon the relief community imposes an obligation both to provide help and to learn how to improve the quality of that help. It is hard to think of any other human setting in which the ethical burden of research is as great. (Leaning 2001, p. 1433)

A parallel argument has been made in medical education, for example, when we claim that the only way medical students can learn would be to practice on patients, and thus there is an ethical obligation to use patients to improve care and assist future patients.

8.2 Disasters and Research Ethics

Less enthusiastic investigators, however, while acknowledging the constraints and difficulties of doing research in time of disaster, recognise that 'disasters rarely constitute an ideal environment to conduct research ... [They] are the most chaotic, stressful and dangerous environments imaginable for doing ... clinical research on human beings' (Bohannon 2011, pp. 1261–1263). Investigators may rush to a disaster site and embark on a research project which has not been fully developed and properly reviewed for its scientific and ethical merit. Procedures may be hastily applied, and protocol transgression may seem justified by the goal of improving future responses and saving lives. Yet, the research could be added onto already burdened humanitarian rescuers, and this added burden could cause additional harm to the research subjects, those who need the most immediate help and support, thus endangering rather than saving lives.

Obtaining a more nuanced and objective view of "disaster research" is complicated. Disasters are multiple and unpredictable; they each have their own peculiar dynamics. As the March 2011 earthquake-tsunami disaster in Japan illustrates, disasters are "uncharted territory" and cannot be effectively managed through traditional survival strategies, routine procedures and stockpiled resources. They create formidable challenges to the community of nations, and nongovernmental organisations (NGOs) that come to the rescue. Even countries like Japan, which are best prepared to manage disasters and boast to be among the nations with the most towering seawalls and the sturdiest buildings in the world, are not immune from the chaos of disasters. Mismanagement in the evacuation process, miscommunication between private and public agencies, and irresponsible conduct of those in charge of the rescue are not uncommon. For example, the rescuers in Japan in the aftermath of the 2011 earthquake and tsunami disaster abandoned survivors to die of starvation (Tabuchi 2012), and allegations were made that doctors in New Orleans euthanized patients during the 2005 Hurricane Katrina (Fink 2009).

Facts on the ground (number of deaths, nature of injuries, and the extent of destruction) rarely fall in line with predictions based on theories. Not all health hazards exacerbate human misery or create health problems; not all disasters are catastrophic or equally tragic. And there is the question of logistics, the day to day, hour to hour, even minute to minute disaster relief responses. Choices must be made between competing evils and be flexible. Disaster victims may qualify as a vulnerable population, although they have not been explicitly recognised as such in any research guidelines or regulations. We must therefore ask whether current research guidelines are applicable to research on victims of disasters.

8.2.1 Risk-benefit Assessments

Among the key ethical requirements for conducting biomedical research are informed consent of subjects and a favourable harm-benefit profile (Emanuel 2000). Research ethics requires that informed consent of subjects is obtained and that the anticipated benefits justify the harms or the risks (of harm) done to research subjects. Harms or risks (of harm) must not outweigh the benefits to be expected from the research. Both requirements—informed consent and a favourable harm/benefit ratio—are necessary for the ethical conduct of human research, but neither alone is sufficient. These requirements are mutually complementary and of equal value: they form a "perfect union." *In practice*, however, it is a real challenge to give these requirements equal value, particularly in disaster research because all of the benefits are to people in the future, i.e., the victims of future similar disasters, and all of the harms or "risks" are to current disaster victims who are used as research subjects, and who may not be in a realistic position to give their informed consent to the research.

In exploring these many challenges I will concentrate on biomedical research on humans because it is the kind of research towards which most guidelines and regulations are directed. I will examine how a utilitarian calculus of harm-benefit assessment plays out when research is done in the wake of a disaster and assess whether such a calculus is sufficient to justify using disaster victims as subjects in clinical trials.

It is worth noting here that the assessment of harm and benefit of research is not a purely objective exercise but is rather a "mix" of facts and values, i.e. the fact of the actual harm done to people right now, and the value that is, at once, attached to this fact (e.g., is the harm worth taking in light of the benefit?) by those making the assessment. This harm-benefit assessment becomes ambiguous and confusing when the concepts of "harm" and "risk" (of harm) are used interchangeably, as it is in most existing research guidelines, and by many investigators and ethics review board members. This is because the term "harm" is not to be understood in probabilistic term, while the notion of "risk" (of harm) is. (The conceptual nature of risks is the product of *both* probability, a scientific notion, and magnitude of harm, a subjective concept)). In making a *risk*-benefit assessment, investigators and institutional review boards (IRBs) would have to decide whether to "gamble" or "play it safe." That this may be a challenging "gamble" at all times, but particularly in time of disaster, simply underlines the difficulties faced by IRBs (also called research ethics committees) in doing a "risk-benefit" or "harm-benefit" assessment themselves.

Moreover, to use disaster victims as subjects in clinical research seems ethically suspect because disasters have their greatest impact on already marginalised and impoverished populations. Yet, the increasing number of disasters worldwide, together with the professionalization of disaster responders and humanitarian organisations, has accelerated the attention paid to what has been labelled a new category of research, 'disaster research', not dealt with in existing codes of research ethics. The need to articulate an ethical justification for this new category of research has also grown, and has gathered momentum in humanitarian and human rights circles where it has been recognised that existing ethics rules do not take into account the status of disaster victims. This book, and the conference on which it is based, is just one example of this recognition.

It seems uncontroversial to conclude that the first (ethical) duty of all humanitarian responders in the immediate *response* phase to a disaster is to provide the victims with the services they need to survive and continue to live decently. Doing clinical research on victims in life-endangering situations runs the risk of ignoring the plight of people caught in disasters. This is because once a favourable benefit-harm ratio is made by an ethics review panel, investigators may be encouraged to focus on possible future benefits to future disasters. As a consequence, the goal of meeting the immediate needs of disaster victims could be seen as nonessential, and informed consent itself may be marginalised, because an independent decision has been made that the research is valuable based on a favourable risk-benefit analysis (Roberts 2011; Boylan 2011; Epstein and Wilson 2011).

8.3 "Big Tent" Research

8.3.1 Epidemiological Research

Research on human beings commonly falls into two main categories: epidemiological and interventional. Epidemiological research, by and large, applies non-invasive data collection methods, e.g., interviews, surveys, focus groups, questionnaires and other similar methodologies, to activities related to quality improvement, education programs, risk exposure, disease surveillance, and the determinants of health.

Although not necessarily risk free (disclosure of confidential or embarrassing information is their main risk), epidemiological research is the least controversial because it is not intrusive, and poses no physical harms to those who consent to participate (Miller and Emanuel 2008). This kind of research generally focuses on improving performance, safety and promoting the health of people right now. It constitutes an integral part of public health activities, and thus is best described as public health practice rather than medical research. The most well-known and foundational example is John Snow's collection of data on the sources of drinking water during a major cholera epidemic in 19th century London. No one was put at risk by his data collection research, and it eventually led to ending the cholera disaster when he identified the source of contaminated drinking water through interpreting his data. Similar epidemiological research, which included accurate and wide sharing of scientific and medical information with both the public and public health professionals was used to identify the source of the Severe Acute Respiratory Syndrome (SARS) epidemic (Kahn 2003).

Epidemiological activities are on-going (e.g. global health surveillance, population movement) and often intensify in complex disasters. The complexity may be related to both the multidimensional aspect of a disaster, and the multifaceted emergency responses it may elicit—responses which themselves may be complicated by the precarious situations of disaster victims. For example, internally displaced persons or refugees may be forced to live in temporary camps in foreign countries because they have been victimised by their home country, or by those they are fighting against in their own country, and may be denied human rights protection generally afforded individuals by treaties, covenant, and international human rights law and ethics.

Documentation of the impact of a disaster on a refugee population has been used to ramp up pressure on the international community to act. In *Nowhere to Turn: Failure to Protect, Support and Assure Justice for Darfur Women*, Physicians for Human Rights (PHR) documented rape, violence and other atrocities suffered by Darfur women in Chad-Sudan border refugee camps. The data they collected and published led to new strategies to try to prevent further assaults on women, meet the immediate needs of women, and plan for their (and their families) safe return to Darfur (PHR 2009).

Médecins Sans Frontières (MSF) describes their own data collection practices (e.g., population surveys, incidence/prevalence risk factor studies) as 'operational research,' emphasising 'interventions' that are readily actionable (and not simply possible or potential). Operational research 'can be annexed to routine operations . . . [and] are likely to have a direct impact on policy and practice and the quality of assistance [MSF] renders to populations' (MSF 2010, p. 9). As we move towards more complex studies (e.g. clinical trials), the greater the likelihood that the research will infringe upon routine operations. As a result, and because of the considerable resources and time required, 'involvement in clinical trials will likely be an exception for MSF' (MSF 2010, p. 9). Instead, by focusing on data collection activities, which can be categorised as epidemiological research, MSF believes it can directly contribute to improving program design and practices and the quality of MSF assistance provided. This kind of activity is analogous to "health services research" which collects data for quality improvement in the delivery of healthcare. In epidemiological or public health activities, including health services research, the risk of harm to people is minimal, and the benefit to others may be great and readily actionable.

8.3.2 Interventional Research

Clinical or interventional biomedical research contrasts sharply with epidemiological data-collection activities in that it uses a protocol and a specific design (e.g., placebo-controlled, randomised) to test a new drug, device or treatment strategy which will predictably cause actual harm to some human beings. Biomedical or behavioural in nature, interventional research is a kind of research at which almost all existing ethical guidelines and regulations are directed, including, of course, the foundational Nuremberg Code, and the Declaration of Helsinki.

The ethical requirements for such research are summarised in the 1976 US code of federal regulations (CFR), modelled after the Nuremberg Code and the *Declaration of Helsinki*, which requires a comprehensive review of the research protocol by an "ethics board" or institutional review board (IRB) before investigators are authorised to approach individuals to ask them whether they want to enrol in the research. IRB approval is based on a number of factors, including a determination that the study is scientifically sound, that the methods employed are appropriate, and, most important for this chapter, that the harm to subjects does not outweigh the anticipated benefits of the research. The study must not begin before individual consent is obtained, even when all other required conditions are met. These requirements are based on fundamental ethical principles of respect for persons and doing no harm. Another ethical principle, beneficence (or doing good), directs the investigator to maximise benefits and minimise harms, and this is usually translated into the requirement of a favourable risk-benefit ratio, the lack of which would invalidate most research on human beings (Wendler 2005).

Looking at the unique research opportunities presented by disasters, together with the reasonable predication that disasters will continue to occur and research may help us gain greater knowledge on how to respond to future disasters, some have even argued that it would be ethically unacceptable not to embrace this opportunity to learn how to improve the care afforded (future) disaster victims and "save lives." The central question, of course, is whether this type of research should be done at all. As I have already suggested, answering this question requires a determination of whether it is possible to objectively evaluate the risks and benefits of proposed disaster research, and whether it is realistic to expect that the disaster victims can provide voluntary informed consent. Before attempting to answer these questions it is useful to provide a brief overview of existing research guidelines and regulations as this may help to suggest the answers.

8.4 Making Sense of Guidelines and Regulations

Informed consent has been first, foremost and central to research on human beings at least since World War II when in 1947 US judges, sitting in judgment of the Nazi doctors at Nuremberg, articulated a set of ten rules which became known as the Nuremberg Code (Shuster 1997). By putting informed consent first, the US judges—who believed they were articulating international law—hoped they could compel future investigators to remain focused on the rights and welfare of their individual subjects who bear the burden and harm of research and need human rights protection (Shuster 1998).

The *first* Rule, 'The voluntary consent of the human subject is absolutely essential,' insists on obtaining voluntary, competent, informed and understanding consent, and also requires that the research subject have sufficient and sufficiently reliable information about 'all inconveniences and hazards reasonably to be expected, and [about] the effects upon his health or person which may possibly come from his participation in the experiment.' Thus, embedded in the informed consent process is a requirement to inform subjects of the risks of harms and potential benefits to be expected from the experiments. The Nuremberg Code has nine additional requirements, the most challenging of which are those that directly relate to the harm-benefit ratio (Nuremberg Code 1949):

> Rule 2. The experiment should be such as to yield fruitful results for the good of society, unprocurable by other methods or means of study, and not random and unnecessary in nature;
> Rule 4. The experiment should be so conducted as to avoid all unnecessary physical and mental suffering and injury;
> Rule 5. No experiment should be conducted where there is an *a priori* reason to believe that death or disabling injury will occur, except, perhaps, in those experiments where the experimental physicians also serve as subjects;
> Rule 6. The degree of risk to be taken should never exceed that determined by the humanitarian importance of the problem to be solved by the experiment.
> Rule 7. Proper preparations should be made and adequate facilities provided to protect the experimental subject against even remote possibilities of injury, disability, or death.
> Rule 10. During the course of the experiment the scientist in charge must be prepared to terminate the experiment at any stage, if he has probable cause to believe, in the exercise of the good faith, superior skill, and careful judgment required of him, that a continuation of the experiment is likely to result in injury, disability, or death to the experimental subject.

Seven of the ten Rules in the Code are relevant to the harm-benefit ratio of research, the assessment of which is done by the subjects (Rule 1) and the investigators (Rules 2, 4–7, 10). This is important because, taken together, these rules establish a balance between the importance given to informed consent (Rule 1), on the one hand, and the importance given to harm or risk-benefit assessment (Rules 2, 4–7,10), on the other hand. In short, both informed consent and a favourable risk-benefit ratio are necessary. Recently, international instruments have adopted the harm-benefit rules to supplement the informed consent requirement, e.g., the 1997 UNESCO *Universal Declaration on the Human Genome and Human Rights* (Article 10), the 1997 *European Convention on Human Rights and Biomedicine* (Article 2) and the 2005 UNESCO *Universal Declaration on Bioethics and Human Rights* (Article 3.2).

The 1964 *Declaration of Helsinki*, Ethical Principles for Medical Research Involving Human Subjects, under the auspices of the World Medical Association (WMA), revised eight times since, has emphasised the primacy of the human being over society, and has appealed to the notion of respect for persons and human dignity. (A similar statement is found in the *Universal Declaration on Bioethics and Human Rights*, Article 3.2.) In spite of its multiple revisions, the 2008 *Declaration of Helsinki* kept intact the language that gives priority to the interests and well-being of individual subjects over all other interests, a language that embodies the core values of all research on human beings (Solbakk 2011). For example, its Introduction reads: 'In medical research involving human subjects, the well-being of the individual research subject must take precedence over all other interests' (WMA 2008, A.6).

The *Declaration* further expanded on a number of relevant ethical principles:

> Principle 17. Medical research involving a disadvantaged or vulnerable population or community is only justified if the research is responsive to the health needs and priorities of this population or community and if there is a reasonable likelihood that this population or community stands to benefit from the results of the research.
> Principle 18. Every medical research study involving human subjects must be preceded by *careful assessment of predictable risks and burdens to the individuals and communities involved in the research in comparison with foreseeable benefits to them and to other individuals or communities affected by the condition under investigation* (emphasis added).
> Principle 20. Physicians may not participate in a research study involving human subjects unless they are confident that *the risks involved have been adequately assessed and can be satisfactorily managed.* Physicians must immediately stop a study when the risks are found to outweigh the potential benefits or when there is conclusive proof of positive and beneficial results (emphasis added).
> Principle 21. Medical research involving human subjects may only be conducted if the importance of the objective outweighs the inherent risks and burdens to the research subjects.
> Principle 24. In medical research involving competent human subjects, each potential subject must be adequately informed of the aims, methods, sources of funding, any possible conflicts of interest, institutional affiliations of the researcher, the *anticipated benefits and potential risks of the study and the discomfort it may entail*, and any other relevant aspects of the study. ... After ensuring that the potential subject has understood the information, the physician or another appropriately qualified individual must then seek the potential subject's freely-given informed consent, preferably in writing ... (WMA 2008; emphasis added)

Nonetheless, it is difficult to envision how these principles could be effectively applied and be actionable in time of disaster when people are vulnerable and socioeconomically distressed. More troublesome are on-going attempts to comply better with the macro-level interests of science and society at the expense of the micro-level interests of individual subjects and their communities. 'Consequently, the quest and striving for a universal normative language in international research also seems to be a morally and legally justifiable endeavour' (Solbakk 2011, p. 342).

The *Declaration of Helsinki* introduces a distinction between "therapeutic (or clinical) research" where the risks of harm are assumed by subjects for their own benefit, and "nontherapeutic (or scientific) research" where the risks of harm are assumed by subjects for the benefit of science and society. As will be discussed later, to combine medical care with medical research complicates the validity of informed consent and compromises the risk-benefit calculation, including the delicate balance that exists between risks taken for one's own benefits and risks taken for the benefit of others (Shuster 1998).

The World Health Organization (WHO)-sponsored *International Ethical Guidelines for Biomedical Research Involving Human Subjects* published in 1993 and since revised by the Council for International Organizations of Medical Science (CIOMS) in 2002 restated the requirement of a favourable harm-benefit ratio and added two points in the context of research done in developing countries.

1. The research project must be responsive to the health conditions or needs of vulnerable subjects. Harm is more easily justified when it arises from interventions that hold out the prospect of direct benefit for the subject population. Harm that does not hold out such a prospect must be justified;
2. In order for the research to be ethical and not exploitive in this setting, it must offer the potential of actual benefit to the people in the developing country in which the research is done.

The WHO *Handbook for Good Clinical Research Practice* (2002), an adjunct to the WHO *Guidelines for Good Clinical Practice (GCP) for Trials on Pharmaceutical Products* (1995), reaffirms the importance of evaluating the benefits and risks of research by institutional review boards, in these terms:

> Principle 3. Before research involving humans is initiated, foreseeable risks and discomforts and any anticipated benefit(s) for the individual trial subject and society should be identified. Research of investigational products or procedures should be supported by adequate non-clinical and, when applicable, clinical information.
> Principle 4. Research involving humans should be initiated only if the anticipated benefits for the individual research subject and society clearly outweigh the risks. *Although the benefit of the results of the trial to science and society should be taken into account, the most important considerations are those related to the rights, safety, and well-being of the trial subjects.* (emphasis added)

It is worth noting here that Principle 4 is the very principle enunciated by the *Declaration of Helsinki* (Introduction A.6) which represents the "normative bedrock" of clinical research involving human beings. However, putting IRBs in charge of getting the best deal for consenting research subjects (through harm-benefit evaluation) and as "gatekeepers" of the entire human research enterprise runs the risk of turning upside down the values expressed in this principle to fit with the interests of the two most powerful players in the field: science and society (Maschke 2008; Solbakk 2011).

Both the 1947 *Nuremberg Code* and the 1964 *Declaration of Helsinki* served as models for the 1976 *US Code of Federal Regulations for the Protection of Human Research Subjects* (CFR 1976) and the 1991 'Common Rule' which applies these regulations across US federal agencies. These Regulations (since revised) utilise the concept of "risk" (of harm) rather than "harm" since the assumption is that almost no research protocol is ethically acceptable if actual harm is to be done to research subjects as part of the protocol. Approval of a research protocol by the Institutional Review Board (IRB) or ethic review panel depends on such assessment. IRBs must therefore find that:

1. *Risks* [of harm] to subjects are *minimized*;
2. *Risks* [of harm] to subjects are *reasonable* in relation to anticipated benefits, if any, to subjects, and the importance of the knowledge that may reasonably be expected to result. (CFR 1976, emphasis added)

Minimum risk should mean that 'the probability and magnitude of harm or discomfort anticipated in the research are not greater, in and of themselves, than those ordinarily encountered in daily life, or during the performance of routine physical or psychological examinations or tests' (CFR 2009). It is also stated that, in evaluating risks and benefits of research, 'the IRB should consider only those risks and benefits that may result from the research (as distinguished from risks and benefits of therapies subjects would receive even if not participating in the research). The IRB should *not* consider possible long-range effects of applying knowledge gained in the research (for example, the possible effects of the research on public policy) as among those research risks that fall within the purview of its responsibility' (CFR 2009).

Excluding long-term risks of research is troublesome and misguided in any research condition, but it is more so in time of disaster because the benefits are almost always in the future and valued in probabilistic terms as part of the harm-benefit assessment, and the risks are always actual and immediate. Not considering the long-term risk effects of research on individuals and society probably makes for an easier risk-benefit calculation, but not for an inclusive, complete and meaningful evaluation.

New ethics guidelines for research in disaster conditions have also been suggested (WHO 1999; Maschke 2008). In 1997, WHO and the *Macfarlane Burnet Center for Medical Research* facilitated an advisory group whose mandate included articulating an ethics framework for research in emergencies, essentially to provide guidance on issues related to risk-benefit and informed consent. This group produced an Ethics Template addressing several areas of ethical concern. The section on risk-benefit reads:

1. The benefit derived from the research must accrue directly and temporally to the actual subjects of the research.
2. The research must be directed at questions that could not be answered in a non-emergency or non-refugee setting.
3. The risks to the individual subjects, their community, and their future security must be kept to an absolute minimum. These risks must be extensively and comprehensively detailed in the research protocol and also *embedded in the protocol for obtaining informed consent.* All anticipated risks should be identified and mechanisms described to monitor for adverse outcomes. A threshold must be defined for intervention and, if needed, interruption of the study. Mechanisms to treat those in whom adverse outcomes develop must be described. The feedback methods by which this monitoring system will be operationalized must be described. (Advisory Group 1997, emphasis added)

The group recognised that some research addresses questions that cannot be answered in nonemergency settings, and that adhering to research ethics principles may be challenging when research is done on people who may be entirely dependent on external aid for their survival. Nonetheless, the advisory group concluded that these challenges should not discourage conducting research during complex emergencies. It was also argued that it could be unethical to avoid carrying out certain relevant research in complex emergencies (WHO 1997). For example, it was suggested that it would be unethical not to conduct research on children who face malnutrition as a result of a disaster. Disaster conditions provide a unique opportunity to learn and gain knowledge on how to improve nutrition and manage malnutrition in these unique environments. Missing this opportunity and not doing such research which could save the lives of children in future disasters could be inherently unethical. Of course, nutritional research can be done, but it should be done on non-vulnerable populations who are not dependent on physician-researchers for their very survival.

One important ethical guideline that applies to all research is that vulnerable groups (such as disaster victims) should almost never be enrolled in research that can be done on non-vulnerable populations. This has also been the conclusion of the *President's Advisory Committee on the Human Radiation Experiments* in the United States. The Committee condemned the use of vulnerable, institutionalised children for research on nutritional studies comparing breakfast cereals—because the study could have been done on non-vulnerable, free-living children, such as the children of the researchers from Massachusetts Institute of Technology (Advisory Committee on Human Radiation Experiments 1995).

8.5 Doing Good in Disaster Research

The difficulty, of course, is to develop a research protocol applicable to disaster conditions that not only values disaster victims, but also values both the requirement of informed consent and the requirement of an ethical harm-benefit ratio. To obtain a voluntary informed consent in any circumstance is extraordinarily difficult, time consuming and costly, when done right. This is more so with disaster research in which a modified "therapeutic illusion" seems inherent (also called the 'philanthropic misconception'). For example, disaster victims will assume what they are told, that the physician-rescuer is there to help them, and not to use them for their own research purposes. This belief (illusion) invalidates informed consent. To the extent that it exists, it also makes a harm-benefit assessment by the subject (regardless of the IRB's assessment) unrealistic—since the subject's assumption is that the intervention is being done to benefit the disaster victim now, not for the benefit of future disaster victims only.

By introducing a distinction between therapeutic and nontherapeutic research, the *Declaration of Helsinki* has done a disservice to research subjects since it reinforces this illusion by confusing the distinction between treatment and research. It permits a different threshold of acceptability of harm for therapeutic research, and thus a more favourable harm-benefit analysis, which is incorrect (Rid and Wendler 2011). Jay Katz, a renowned psychiatrist and expert on informed consent, insisted on the vital importance of maintaining the distinction between research and therapy, and deplored its blurring in practice. Not making a clear distinction between research and treatment also blurs the distinction between physician and researcher, and between patient and research subject. Without a clear understanding that they are in research, people tend to believe that their personal interests and not science's, are being served (Katz 1993). Researchers follow a protocol to gain new knowledge from research subjects; research is not treatment done for the benefit of individual patients. The fiduciary relationship between doctors and patients fundamentally differs from the research relationship between investigators and subjects.

Disaster victims need help and treatment. They do not seek or desire to be subjects in a research project that holds risks but no benefits for them. Moreover, disaster conditions make it unlikely that victims will be able to give voluntary and informed consent or to make an independent harm-benefit assessment of any proposed clinical research. To approve the research protocol, the IRB must have found the harm-benefit assessment favourable. Therefore the protocol comes to the field with an embedded presumption that some "good" may come from the research, if not now, in the future. To obtain these benefits, however, the research must be done: giving a motivation to "sell" the research to the potential subject, a natural tendency that undermines the consent process itself. In this context, the harm-benefit trade-off, which presumably should protect subjects in research, is likely to provide little or no protection.

8.6 Minimising Risks of Harm

The US Federal Regulations state that risks to subjects must be minimal, "reasonable," or not "excessive," compared to potential benefits. Jennifer Leaning specifies that studies should impose 'the absolute minimum of additional risk' (Leaning 2001, p. 1432). However, there is no agreed-on definition of what "minimal" risk should be. For example, the *Additional Protocol to the Convention on Human Rights and Biomedicine, concerning Biomedical Research* 'deemed that the research bears a minimal risk if, having regard to the nature and scale of the intervention, it is to be expected that it will result, at the most, in a very slight and temporary negative impact on the health of the person concerned' (Council of Europe 2005, Article 17). The CIOMS Guidelines hold that 'the risk from research interventions that do not hold out the prospect of direct benefit for the individual subject [lacking decision making capacity] should be no more likely and not greater than the risk attached to routine medical or psychological examination of such persons' (CIOMS 2002, Guideline 9). As noted previously, Federal Research Regulations define "minimal risk" as 'the amount of risk ordinarily encountered in daily life.' These definitions, however, are problematic.

Harm may be serious (magnitude of harm), and yet viewed as minimal because the probability of it occurring is extremely low, or conversely, it can be minimal and yet viewed as serious because the probability of it occurring is very high. This assessment may also be affected by its relation to benefits, whether they are present or future. To compare minimal risk to those risks "ordinarily encountered in daily life" is not useful because many daily life activities may include risks that are unacceptably high, particularly in time of disasters, and this could justify doing all kinds of research, even the most bizarre and fanciful.

The term "benefit" is no less problematic and controversial because the concept is given a positive value attached to future benefit, such as potentially improving the health and welfare of people in the future. But in Phase I clinical trials there are no expected benefits to subjects—Phase I is, by definition and purpose, a nontherapeutic, phase to determine safety. The main question in Phase I trials often boils down to this: 'what level (or magnitude) of harm should a subject be allowed to withstand in the name of research?' (Shamoo and Resnik 2003, p. 194). Harm is expected to be immediate (i.e., in drug trials, dosage is increased incrementally until it harms the subject—hopefully minimally). Only a comprehensive informed consent regimen and a rigid monitoring protocol to minimise harm can justify a Phase I trial. But neither informed consent nor strict and careful monitoring of the research protocol seems likely in the immediate aftermath of a disaster. And it is difficult to envision how individuals caught in a disaster may "benefit from the fruits of research" (as suggested by CIOMS guidelines) either because disaster victims may have moved elsewhere and could not be located, have died or because research results have been too long coming, therefore no longer relevant, or if still relevant have not been made readily available to them. Requiring that subjects and beneficiaries of research are of the same group makes most research in disaster settings ethically untenable.

Research rules in ordinary settings are now being reconsidered in the United States, particularly, the cost-benefit assessment of applying the current research regulations themselves. One common belief is that current regulations impose burdensome bureaucratic procedures on researchers that do little to enhance effectiveness, protect research participants and reduce costs (Emanuel 2011). These regulations frustrate researchers who may be prevented or significantly delayed from doing valuable research that could "save lives" (Whitney and Schneider 2011; Holm 2011). However, improving research efficiency by reducing the cost of research and eliminating burdensome regulations has less to do with ethics than with economics. Efficiency is an economic goal; it is not an ethical principle.

Arguably, cost-benefit analysis is like risk-benefit assessment: it is about process and efficiency, and not about actually protecting the rights of subjects in research. It is about a determination by the IRB that the proportionality of foreseeable harm and potential benefit is (or is not) favourable and that risks of harm to subjects are in proportion to (and balanced by) the expected benefits (to subjects or others). Although statistical assessments are empirical or scientific, the evaluation of harms and benefits are value judgments made by those making the assessments. In clinical drug trials on healthy or diseased subjects, for example, harm to subjects is expected to be immediate and actual—and hopefully minimal—and IRBs must speculate about future benefits to subjects (if any) and to society (usually in non-probabilistic terms, and in a pro forma manner). In this context, IRBs' pronouncements may not stand serious scrutiny since the data necessary to arrive at a valid risk-benefit evaluation are usually unavailable—and can emerge only if the research project is in fact done.

8.7 Prisoners of Disasters

It is unremarkable that would-be researchers largely expect that "good" will come from their work. But this is not evidence-based reasoning which anyone, including IRBs should take seriously. Investigators and IRB members must do better if the goal is to demonstrate that biomedical research in the immediate aftermath of a disaster can be done ethically, while protecting the rights and welfare of subjects. A comparison with prisoners, a vulnerable population, may be useful. Like prisoners, disaster victims (especially, but not only, those in refugee camps) may have lost their freedom of movement and become dependent on others for everything, including food, medicine and basic essentials. In this regard, because of the fear and danger inherent in disaster settings, victims of disaster are likely to be an even more vulnerable population than prisoners when it comes to proposals to do research on them.

In his *Acres of Skin: Human Experimentation in Holmesburg Prison,* Allen Hornblum underlines the effects of disasters (specifically, World War II) on human experimentation in America. 'It was during the war years that the federal prison system swung into action as a major source of human subjects for research experiments ... Prisoners were too valuable as research subjects to be jettisoned. They needed to be used, not protected' (Hornblum 1998, pp. 83, 85). Sociology Professor David Rothman, commenting on this time of transformation, explained that 'a utilitarian ethic continued to govern human experimentation—partly because of the war precedent, partly because the benefits seemed so much greater than the costs, and partly, too, because there were no groups or individuals prominently opposing such an ethic' (Rothman 1987, p. 1198).

The 1976 Report of the National Commission for the Protection of Human Subjects in Biomedical and Behavioral Research permits research on prisoners only in limited circumstances. The Commission focused on two key ethical considerations: '(1) whether prisoners bear a fair share of the burdens and receive a fair share of the benefits of research [i.e. harm-benefit assessment]; and (2) whether prisoners are, in the words of the Nuremberg Code, "so situated as to be able to exercise free power of choice"—that is, whether prisoners can give *truly voluntary consent* to participate in research' (1976, p. 5, emphasis added). It found that prison was no place to conduct biomedical and behavioural research because prisoners are in a setting that makes it impossible for them to freely and voluntarily consent to participate.

The Institute of Medicine (IOM) was asked to review this position to determine whether it is justified today. Using a utilitarian ethics, the IOM Committee questioned the weight placed on informed consent and on prisoners' status and concluded that current restrictions on using prisoners in biomedical and behavioural research should be loosened and the overall oversight boosted (IOM 2006). The Committee made a number of recommendations, the most telling of which was advising a shift from a *category-based* to a *risk-benefit* approach to research review.

Commenting on this recommendation, Osagie Obasogie, a law professor at the University of California, Los Angeles, perceptively observed that 'shifting from prisoners' almost categorical exclusion from research to a more permissive risk-benefit analysis—is where the ethical road meets the legal rubber' (Obasogie 2010, p. 58). Quoting from the IOM report that states that '[m]ore attention needs to be paid to risks and risk-benefit analysis rather than the formalities of an informed consent document' (IOM 2006, p. 118), Obasogie contends: 'This shapes the major recommendation [of the IOM Committee] to stop thinking of prisoners as a category of individuals who, by default, should not be human subjects.... [and instead] recommends looking at each research proposal on a case-by-case basis to assess its potential risks and benefits' (Obasogie 2010, p. 58). This, Obasogie argues, is a serious ethical mistake. To favour independently weighing risks against benefits to permit more prison research takes the emphasis off the rights and dignity of the individuals who bear the burdens of research, and transfers it to an abstract analysis of harms and benefits by an IRB.

The fatal flaw with the IOM Report is that once the IRB decides that the harm-benefit ratio of the proposed research is favourable, obtaining a valid informed consent from the prisoners can be viewed (and treated) as mechanical and marginal. The fundamental question is no longer *whether* research in prison conditions should be done (and whether a voluntary informed consent can be obtained), but rather *how* this particular research should be done, and informed consent obtained. 'This shift from a *substantive* approach to justice and respect for persons (emphasizing protection, fairness, and burden-sharing) to a more *procedural* mechanism (emphasizing representation, along with the noncategorical risk/benefit analysis)' is where the IOM committee misses the mark (Obasogie 2010, p. 59).

Disaster victims are in many ways like prisoners, and disaster research is, at least in the immediate aftermath of a disaster, like prison research. Although no one has done the research needed to prove the proposition (by examining how IRBs actually review disaster research), I think it makes intuitive sense to believe that just as the IOM envisions harm-benefit analysis taking precedence over informed consent in prison research, this same result is likely in disaster research. This is for at least two reasons. The first reason is that the benefits are almost always overblown and concern future disaster victims, science and the greater society (Zhang 2013). The second reason is that the weaker the interest in improving the informed consent *process,* the stronger the need to provide exhaustive informed consent *forms*, while at the same time complaining that these forms consume too much IRB time, too much energy, too many resources, and are incomprehensible to most research subjects, and therefore useless (Emanuel 2011).

It may be objected that we should not designate "disaster victims" as a new category of vulnerable research subjects because disaster research is critical for progress, and also because a utilitarian ethics (harm-benefit calculus) may be sufficient to protect human subjects from harm. Additional research protection for disaster victims may not only be unnecessary, it may also be counterproductive since it may slow or even stop research pertaining to their situations and could deny future disaster victims the benefits of research. The problem with this stance is that there appears to be no morally defensible reason for thinking that a risk-benefit calculation protects subjects from harm. This is because in this calculation, as previously noted, the benefits of research are always potential and speculative, i.e., for people in the future, and the risk of harm is always definite, actual and immediate, i.e. for people right now. Long-term potential harms to subjects are generally ignored or overlooked. In short, weighing the risk-benefit ratio of research on human beings may not promote subjects' protection and may add to the pitfalls inherent to the utilitarian calculation noted above.

8.8 "Saving Lives"

The powerful "saving lives" mantra is the core justification for doing research in disaster condition (Annas 2010). This rationale by investigators is, however, almost entirely self-serving, very much like the argument pharmaceutical companies make to justify the high price of their products to fund research on new products that might benefit people in the future. But people who are injured and traumatised by a disaster need treatment right now (Zhang 2013). Just as pharmaceutical companies have a moral obligation to sell their products at a price people who need them can afford, so too first responders and humanitarian workers have a moral obligation to provide immediate relief and help to people in distress without adding to their burdens and affliction.

Humanitarian and human rights physician, Paul Farmer, observed in the aftermath of Paul Duvalier's violent and dictatorial regime:

> In Haiti, research was not a part of what Haitians have hoped for ... Research did not figure on the wish list of the people we were trying to serve. Services are what they asked for, and as people who had been displaced by political and economic violence, they regarded these services as rightful remedies for what they had suffered. (Farmer 2005, p. 205)

Disasters create health and human rights problems which investigators, IRBs and the entire human research enterprise are ill equipped to address: 'in human rights work, research and critical assessment are insufficient—analysis alone cannot curb human rights violations ...' (Farmer 2005, p. 205).

The 2011 earthquake-tsunami disaster in Japan demonstrates that there is plenty of room for disaster-related research activities, but none that I have been able to identify justify doing biomedical research on human beings in its immediate aftermath. For example, research is justified and even necessary to improve earthquake proofing of buildings for people living in earthquake prone countries. Such research is on buildings and is not on people and can be an important part of disaster planning (or Emergency Management) in prevention, preparedness, and recovery phases. Likewise, evaluating the benefit of seawalls as a first line of defence against tsunamis is necessary, but this research is not done on human beings; it is done on seawalls. Like scientific investigators, structural engineers may legitimately claim that they are "saving lives" by experimenting on how best to secure buildings immediately after a destructive earthquake (recovery phase). But, in the response phase of an emergency, they are obligated to do what they know best to manage damages and contain human casualties. There is no ethically appropriate research that cannot be done before a disaster or after disaster conditions have been addressed and people are out of danger.

Epidemiological research, including monitoring the radiation exposure of disaster victims, and keeping track of them for years, even decades, to see what doses caused what diseases, is perfectly reasonable. This kind of disaster research is *not* to be compared to the highly controversial "emergency research" which the US Food and Drug Administration (FDA) approved without informed consent on unconscious out-of-hospital heart attack or automobile accident victims with life-threatening injuries for which no good medical treatments existed (FDA 1996).

8.9 Summary

"Disaster research" is a new category of research that could rapidly expand. In this chapter I have argued that epidemiological research conducted by investigators or public health professionals in time of a disaster (i.e. in the response phase to a disaster) is both reasonable and necessary. Survey, data collection, questionnaire-type activities which do not add burdens onto people affected by a disaster and/or create obstacles to their being helped and treated, is reasonable and necessary; so too it is reasonable and necessary to assess "life safety" or security of those who flee their homes to find refuge in refugee camps. These activities are an integral part of public health practices which aim at helping people right now and improving their security, health and wellbeing. They are done in the interests of disaster victims, directly related to their immediate needs. Benefits are not secured at the cost of inflicting additional harms to disaster victims (though nothing in life is risk free) or at the cost of exploiting people for our purposes.

By contrast, biomedical research conducted in the immediate aftermath of a disaster is *not* in the interests of disaster victims. Disaster conditions are usually so dire that they create an obligation to categorise disaster victims as "vulnerable" and as a category of individuals who, like prisoners, need more, rather than less, protection from exploitation. Put another way, disasters create no exception to the ethical rules or human rights principles that govern biomedical research on human beings.

Debate, however, will undoubtedly continue and questions will be raised about whether ethics guidelines and regulations should be relaxed or waived to permit more research in disaster settings to "save lives." The great American novelist, F. Scott Fitzgerald, gave an impressive portrayal of Americans and American culture when he wrote at the end of *The Great Gatsby,* 'Gatsby believed in the green light, the orgiastic future that year by year recedes before us. It eluded us then, but that's no matter—tomorrow we will run faster, stretch out our arms farther . . . And one fine morning—So we beat on, boats against the current, born back ceaselessly into the past' (Fitzgerald 1925, p. 189).

The research beat will also go on, faster and undoubtedly louder. And it is probably a good thing to believe, like Gatsby, in the 'green light' if we want to improve our lives, make worthwhile discoveries and assert the most basic right to survival. Research is an important human endeavour and may help us achieve these goals, but it is only a means to an end; it cannot (and should not) be an end in itself. This is because the progress that research promises may be too dazzling. It may come at an unacceptably high price, especially once it has been decided that research in the wake of a disaster has enormously vital potential benefits to science and society which could make the actual risks to research subjects marginal, even irrelevant. Hans Jonas, I think, got it right when he wrote about the relationship between progress and research on vulnerable humans 'Progress is an optional goal, not an unconditional commitment, and that its tempo in particular, compulsive as it may become, has nothing sacred about it . . . Too ruthless a pursuit of scientific progress would make its most dazzling triumphs not worth having.' (Jonas 1969, pp. 219–247)

References

Advisory Committee on Human Radiation Experiments. 1995. US Government Printing Office.

Advisory Group on Research in Emergencies. 1997. Annex—Ethics Template. http://apps.who.int/eha/resource/pubs/160499p.htm. Accessed 11 May 2011.

Annas, George J. 2010. *Worst case bioethics. Death, disaster, and public health*. Oxford: Oxford University Press.

Barzilay, Ezra, Nicolas Schaad, Roc Magoire, Kam S. Mung, Jacques Boncy, Georges A. Dahourou, Eric D. Mintz, Maria W. Steenland, John F. Vertefeuille, and Jordan W. Tappero. 2013. Cholera surveillance during Haiti epidemic—The first 2 years. *New England Journal of Medicine* 368:599–609.

Bohannon, Jean. 2011. War as a laboratory for trauma research. *Science* 331:1261–1263.

Boylan, John F, Niamh P. Conton, Mohammad J. Jaigirdar. 2011. Consent in emergency care research. *The Lancet* 378:25.

Code of Federal Regulations (CFR). 1976. 45 CFR 46.

Code of Federal Regulations (CFR). 2009. 45 CFR 46.102 (D).

Council for International Organizations of Medical Science (CIOMS). 2002. International ethical guidelines for biomedical research involving human subjects. http://www.cioms.ch/publications/layout_guide2002.pdf. Accessed 8 June 2013.

Council of Europe. 2005. Additional protocol to the convention on human rights and biomedicine. http://conventions.coe.int/Treaty/en/Treaties/Html/195.htm. Accessed 7 June 2012.

Emanuel, Ezekiel J., and Jerry Menikoff. 2011. Reforming the regulations governing research with human subjects. *New England Journal of Medicine* 365:1145–1150.

Emanuel, Ezekiel J., David Wendler, and Christine Grady. 2000. What makes clinical research ethical? *Journal of the American Medical Association* 283 (20): 2701–11.

Epstein, Mirian, and Mark Wilson. 2011. Consent in emergency care research. *The Lancet* 378:26.

Farmer, Paul. 2005. *Pathologies of power: Health, human rights, and the new war on the poor*, 205. University of California Press.

Fitzgerald, F. Scott. 1925. *The Great Gatsby*. New York: Charles Scribner.

Fink, Sheri. 2009. The deadly choices at Memorial. *New York Times*, 25 Aug.

Food, and Drug Administration (FDA). 1996. Exception from informed consent requirements for emergency research. 21CFR 50.24.

Holm, S. 2011. Commentary: Systems, rules and the costs of being ethical—A response to D. Chalmers and to S. Whitney and C. Schneider. *Journal of Internal Medicine* 269:403–408.

Hornblum, Allen M. 1998. *Acres of skin: Human experiments at Holmesburg prison*. New York: Routledge.

Institute of Medicine (IOM). 2006. *Ethical considerations for research involving prisoners*. Washington, DC: National Academy Press.

Jonas, Hans. 1969. Philosophical reflections on experimenting with human subjects. *Daedalus* 98 (2): 219–247.

Kahn, Jeffrey. 2003. It's a small world after all: Ethics and the response to SARS. *Hastings Center Report* 33 (3): 6.

Katz, Jay. 1993. Ethics and clinical research revisited: A tribute to Henry K. Beecher. *Hastings Center Report* 23 (5): 36.

Largent, Emily A., Steven Joffe, Franklin G. Miller. 2011. Can research and care be ethically integrated? *Hastings Center Report* 41 (4): 37–46.

Leaning, Jennifer. 2001. Ethics of research in refugee populations. *The Lancet* 357:1432–1433.

Maschke, Karen J. 2008. Human research protections: Time for regulatory reform? *Hastings Center Report* 38 (2): 19–22.

Médecins, Sans Frontières (MSF). 2010. Operational research: Definition, purposes and procedures (A policy framework). http://fieldresearch.msf.org/msf/bitstream/10144/190889/1/OR%20Policy%202010.pdf. Accessed 19 June 2013

Miller, Franklin, and Ezekiel Emanuel. 2008. Quality improvement research and informed consent. *New England Journal of Medicine* 358:765–767.
National Commission for the Protection of Human Subjects of Biomedical and Behavioral research. 1976. Report and recommendations: Research involving prisoners. Bethesda. DHEW Publication No. (OS) 76–131.
Nuremberg Code. 1949. http://www.hhs.gov/ohrp/archive/nurcode.html. Accessed 5 June 2013.
Obasogie, Osagie K. 2010. Prisoners as human subjects: A closer look at the Institute of Medicine's recommendations to loosen current restrictions on using prisoners in scientific research. *Stanford Journal of Civil Rights and Civil Liberties* 6 (1): 41–82.
Physician for Human Rights. 2009. Nowhere to turn: Failure to protect, support and assure justice for Darfuri women. https://s3.amazonaws.com/PHR_Reports/nowhere-to-turn.pdf. Accessed 23 June 2013.
Presidential Commission for the Study of Bioethical Issues. 2013. *Safeguarding children. Pediatric medical countermeasure research.* Washington, DC.
Reed, Holly. 2002. *Research ethics in complex humanitarian emergencies. Summary of a Workshop.* Washington, DC: National Academy Press. http://www.nap.edu/catalog/10481.html Accessed 18 June 2013.
Rid, Annette, and David Wendler. 2011. A framework for risk-benefit evaluations in biomedical research. *Kennedy Institute of Ethics Journal* 21 (2): 141–179.
Roberts, Ian, David Pietro-Merino, Haleema Shakur, Iain Chalmers, and Jon Nicholl. 2011. Effect of consent rituals on mortality in emergency care research. *The Lancet* 377:1071–1072.
Rothman, David J. 1987. Ethics and human experimentation: Henry Beecher revisited. *New England Journal of Medicine* 317:1195–1199.
Shamoo, Adil E., and David B. Resnik. 2003. *Responsible conduct of research.* New York: Oxford University Press.
Shuster, Evelyne. 1997. Fifty years later: The significance of the Nuremberg Code. *New England Journal of Medicine* 337:1436–1440.
Shuster, Evelyne. 1998. The Nuremberg Code: Hippocratic ethics and human rights. *The Lancet* 351:974–977.
Solbakk, Jan H. 2011. In the ruins of Babel: Pitfalls on the way toward a universal language for research ethics and benefit sharing. *Cambridge Quarterly of Healthcare Ethics* 20:341–355.
Tabuchi, Hiroko. 2012. An anniversary of 'heartbreaking grief' in Japan. *New York Times*, 11 March. http://www.nytimes.com/2012/03/12/world/asia/a-year-later-effects-of-japans-disaster-are-still-unfolding.html. Accessed 24 June 2013.
Wendler, David. 2005. Protecting subjects who cannot give consent: Toward a better standard for "minimal" risks. *Hastings Center Report* 35 (5): 37–43.
Whitney, Simon N., and Carl E. Schneider. 2011. Viewpoint: A method to estimate the cost in lives of ethics board review of biomedical research. *Journal of Internal Medicine* 269:396–402.
World Health Organization (WHO). 1995. *Guidelines for good clinical practice (GCP) for trials on pharmaceutical products.* http://apps.who.int/prequal/info_general/documents/TRS850/WHO_TRS_850-Annex3.pdf. Accessed 11 June 2013.
World Health Organization (WHO). 1997. Report of consultation on applied health research priorities in complex emergencies. Geneva: WHO.
World Health Organization (WHO). 1999. Applied health research in emergency settings. Document: 12983. http://cidbimena.desastres.hn/docum/crid/Enero2006/CD-2/pdf/eng/doc12983/doc12983.htm. Accessed 11 June 2013.
World Health Organization (WHO). 2002. *Handbook for good clinical research practice (GCP).* http://apps.who.int/prequal/info_general/documents/GCP/gcp1.pdf. Accessed 11 June 2013.
World Medical Association (WMA). 2008. Declaration of Helsinki—ethical principles for medical research involving human subjects 1964. http://www.wma.net.en.30publications.10policies/b3/. Accessed 5 June 2013.
Zhang, Sarah. 2013. Haiyan prompts risk research. *Nature* 503:324.

Chapter 9
Purple Dinosaurs and Victim Consent to Research in Disasters

George J. Annas

> *The voluntary consent of the human subject is absolutely essential.*
>
> Nuremberg Code, 1947

9.1 Introduction

Men Who Stare at Goats, starring George Clooney and Jeff Bridges, was not a major box office smash. That is too bad, because the 2009 movie, based on real events, convincingly portrayed a US military and CIA that is comfortable doing secret, dangerous experiments without consent, and equally adept at making them appear both necessary and harmless when exposed. The use of loud music as part of a torture regime during the early phases of the Iraq war was, for example, portrayed as making prisoners listen to a song sung by Barney the Purple Dinosaur (the lead character in the Public Broadcasting System's (PBS) TV children's show, "Barney and Friends") (Ronson 2004). The pretend child's dinosaur made this form of torture appear trivial and harmless, and it was covered this way in US news outlets. The US military has an unflattering history of research without consent on its troops (Annas 1998; U.S. v. Stanley 1987). Secret CIA research is much more difficult to monitor.

Not to stretch the metaphor beyond recognition, but the trend in civilian medical research has been to try to take the emphasis off of the rights of human subjects, especially the right of (informed) consent and the right to withdraw, and instead place the emphasis on the welfare of society—emphasising the potential benefits of pursuing medical research (Shuster 2013). Under this approach, Institutional Review Boards (IRBs) concentrate on consent forms rather than the consent process, consent is seen as inapplicable or impractical in certain settings, and with impaired populations. More disturbing, in some instances, such as 'emergency research,' consent is seen as not necessary at all—like a pretend purple dinosaur that is nice to have around, but can be discarded as ultimately not critical to the research enterprise (Fost 1998; Guidance 2011). How should consent be treated when research on the victims of a disaster is suggested? Is it ever ethically and legally acceptable to do research on disaster victims, in a disaster setting, without their informed consent? I will argue

G. J. Annas (✉)
Boston University, Boston, USA
e-mail: annasgj@bu.edu

D. P. O'Mathúna et al. (eds.), *Disaster Bioethics: Normative Issues When Nothing is Normal*, Public Health Ethics Analysis 2, DOI 10.1007/978-94-007-3864-5_9,

in this chapter that the answer must be no, and if obtaining the informed consent of disaster victims is impossible, research on this population should simply not be done. Upholding the human rights and human dignity of the current disaster victims is more important than trying to obtain the benefits of research for future disaster victims.

I explain my conclusion by examining post-World War II medical research done without consent. Because it is an excellent case of disaster-related research (in this case justified by war) done without consent, and because it was the subject of a year-long investigation by the U.S. Presidential Commission for the Study of Biomedical Issues, I will use the 1946–48 Guatemala sexually transmitted disease (STD) research studies as a major example to explore the ethical issues raised by research on adults without their consent (Ethically Impossible 2011). I suggest that failure to take consent seriously has led not only to the vicious exploitation of research subjects—especially in disaster-justified research like the Guatemala example, but has also encouraged useless and marginal research with no benefits and significant harms. The CIA's MKULTRA experiments on the effects of LSD on unsuspecting subjects, done during the "disaster" of the Korean War and its aftermath, is the best known of these (Ronson 2004). These secret non-consensual experiments are routinely denounced or marginalised as unauthorised or harmless, but they represent a larger problem: the tendency toward ethical meltdown in international medical research governance which to this day seems to be intent on marginalising informed consent. One method employed is to emphasise the utilitarian values embodied in a utopian view of the societal benefits of research as more important than the deontological values embodied in the human rights and human dignity of research subjects. Another is to convert informed consent from a noun to a verb, as in "to consent the subject," which makes the researcher the active agent, and the subject passive. Still a third is to obliterate the distinction between research and treatment, and use justifications for treatment without consent in a doctor-patient relationship as justifications for doing research without informed consent in a researcher-subject relationship. The central example I use is the series of US-sponsored experiments in Guatemala conducted shortly after World War II, all done without consent in clear violation of the Nuremberg Code, and the political fallout from their revelation more than fifty years later, in 2010 (Reverby 2011; Ethically Impossible 2011).

Guatemala is no stranger to US intrigue. Tim Weiner begins his celebrated history of the CIA, *Legacy of Ashes*, with the first two coups the then-new CIA engineered after World War II: Iran and Guatemala (Weiner 2007). The Guatemala coup is described as a 'turning point in the history of the CIA,' and set at least two precedents. The first was that the CIA 'did not feel bound ... to observe all the ethical rules.' The second, in the words of Senator Mick Mansfield in 1954, was secrecy: 'Secrecy now beclouds everything about the CIA—its cost, its efficiency, its successes, its failures' (Weiner 2007, p. 105). These same observations could be made in relation to the US research in Guatemala. But harsher words have been used, including 'outrageous' (Graniger and Rosenberg 2010), 'shocking' (McNeil 2010), 'reprehensible' (Fox News 2010) and 'appalling ... from a dark chapter in the history of medicine' (Stein 2010). The Presidential Commission agreed with these assessments, concluding that the Guatemala experiments involved 'reprehensible exploitation' that should never be repeated (Ethically Impossible 2011, p. 108).

The targets of these adjectives are the STD experiments in Guatemala from 1946 to 1948 sponsored by the US Public Health Service (PHS), and conducted by a PHS physician who would later take over the Tuskegee syphilis study in the US, John C. Cutler. The research itself was never published and was only brought to light by Tuskegee historian Susan Reverby who came across it in a University of Pittsburgh archive containing Cutler's private papers (Smith 2010). Her own paper on the studies was posted on the internet following public apologies for the research by President Barack Obama, as well as the US Secretary of State, Secretary of Health and Human Services, and head of the National Institutes of Health, as well as pledges to investigate the experiments further (Reverby 2011). With the exception of Tuskegee itself (Jones 1981; Reverby 2000; Reverby 2009) and the Human Radiation Experiments (Advisory Committee 1996) there has never been a similar acknowledgement of the gravity of misuse of human subjects by the American government.

9.2 The Guatemala Experiments

As described by Reverby, and later by the Presidential Commission, the Guatemala experiments were carried out by John Cutler of the PHS and Juan Funes, Guatemala's leading venereal disease public health official. The studies, denoted 'a series of experimental studies on syphilis in man,' were to test the human response to 'fresh infective material [syphilis] to enhance body response to disease . . . ' and 'to find ways to prevent disease immediately after exposure' (Reverby 2011). The human subjects were sex workers, prisoners, children, mental patients, and soldiers. The prisoner studies took place at Guatemala City's Central Penitentiary, which housed approximately 1500 male inmates. In one study, sex workers who tested positive for either syphilis or gonorrhoea were paid to have sex with prisoners. In another, uninfected sex workers had an inoculum of these diseases placed on their cervixes prior to having sex with the prisoners. The prisoners were tested for infection before and after intercourse, and divided into groups to test various chemical agents for prophylaxis. In case of infection, penicillin was provided for cure. Scientific complications with the study included that few men got syphilis, and the blood tests used to confirm syphilis produced many false positives. Doing repeat blood withdrawals produced resistance to continuing to participate in the prisoners, which in turn led the researchers to try to develop a better diagnostic test (Reverby 2011). Although done after World War II, these were fundamentally war-justified experiments. Cutler, for example, argued that 'the purpose was to develop more effective preventative tools for U.S. military personnel' (Ethically Impossible 2011, p. 42). Likewise, his Guatemalan hosts saw the research as disaster-related, with the Chief of the Guatemalan Army Medical Department writing Cutler in June 1947 'beseeching you to draw up an Emergency Venereal Disease

Prophylaxis Plan for (the Military Medical Department), which would be implemented in the National Army as soon as possible' (Ethically Impossible 2011, p. 34).

To try to develop a better diagnostic test the researchers used blood from children, aged 6 to 16, at the National Orphanage (the children were not given syphilis; 89 of 438 gave positive results on their blood test, but had no clinical evidence of disease), because they were unlikely to have been sexually exposed to syphilis. Research using children is always ethically suspect because they cannot consent for themselves, but blood studies like this one were not unusual, and were widely known and routinely published (Stout and Cutler 1951; Funes 1953). It was the third source of research subjects that is perhaps most horrifying: patients in the country's only asylum. The researchers directly inoculated the asylum residents with disease. Cooperation of the facility administrators was obtained by providing drugs and other supplies, and of the subjects by offering them cigarettes. The inoculum of syphilis was applied to the women's bodies on their forearms, face or mouth after they were abraded with needles. In the males, one method was that the penis itself was abraded by scraping it with a hypodermic needle (just short of drawing blood) and then a dressing containing a syphilitic emulsion was applied for one to two hours. Others included scraping the forearm, ingestion of syphilitic material mixed with water, removal of spinal fluid, mixing it with syphilis, and then returning it to the body, and direct injection (Reverby 2011; Ethically Impossible 2011).

CDC Director Thomas Frieden and Francis Collins, Director of the US National Institutes of Health (NIH), have suggested three reasons why these Guatemala studies are especially ethically-problematic: (1) subjects were members of vulnerable populations who could not give valid consent; (2) subjects were intentionally infected with pathogens that could cause serious illness; and (3) deception was used in conducting the experiments (Frieden and Collins 2010). I think they are right about all of these, but I will focus primarily on the consent requirement. Deception, of course, is intimately related to consent, and was also at the core of the Tuskegee experiments. The fact that Cutler was deeply involved in Tuskegee is what both led to the discovery of his Guatemala experiments, and what makes them newsworthy today. Cutler is also perhaps better known for a statement attributed to him by Tuskegee historian James Jones on a PBS television special on Tuskegee. Asked by Jones whether he thought the Nuremberg Doctors' Trial was relevant to his research, Cutler responded, 'No, they were Nazis' (Jones 1981, p. 180). It is worth noting that not only did the Nuremberg Code, enunciated by US judges at the conclusion of the Nazi "Doctors' Trial" at Nuremberg in 1947 (Annas and Grodin 1992), make informed consent mandatory, its consent rule has since been adopted in international law (International Covenant on Civil and Political Rights 1966). The treaty permits no exceptions to the informed consent requirement for medical research, even in an emergency that threatens the very existence of the state, perhaps the ultimate "disaster." Of course, no individual country, no administrative agency (like the US Food and Drug Administration [FDA]), and no group of physicians (such as the World Medical Association), can unilaterally change international law.

9.3 Guatemala in Context

At a press conference called to discuss the Guatemala experiments, Francis Collins underlined the critical importance of informed consent, saying, 'I want to emphasize that today the regulations that govern research funded by the United States government, whether conducted domestically or internationally, would absolutely prohibit this type of study' (Transcript 2010). Asked about 'how many other horrendous ethical abuses like this [Guatemala] might be out there' Collins replied, 'one can identify, and this is in the (United States) published literature, more than 40 other studies where intentional infection was carried out with what we would now consider to be completely inadequate consent . . . ' (Transcript 2010). The NIH later released the citations for these studies. The point seemed to be that the US did not have to go to Guatemala to do secret, unethical research—we were doing the same types of research here in the US. And this is true. The NIH list is a useful catalogue and joins two other well-known lists of ethically questionable studies: those published in Jay Katz's 1972 text on *Experimentation in Humans* (Katz 1972), and those collected in 1966 by Henry Beecher (Beecher 1966).

The publication dates of the 41 intentional-infection studies on the 2010 NIH list range from 1944, two years prior to the Guatemala experiments, to 1981. The majority, 25, used prisoners as research subjects, perhaps the closest analogy to disaster victims, at least when they are geographically trapped by war, earthquake, flooding, or other catastrophe. The published studies encompass a wide range of diseases, including malaria (seven), influenza (five), Norwalk virus (five), hepatitis (eight), respiratory diseases (five), protozoan parasites (four), and even cancer (one). Only three dealt with gonorrhoea or syphilis, and two of these were co-authored by the same John Cutler who presided over the Guatemala study. Both were done in US prisons, one before his Guatemala studies, and one after, and these two studies serve to put the Guatemala work in international ethical context.

In the first study, Cutler and his PHS colleagues sought to study gonorrhoea prophylaxis using as subjects 241 prisoners in the US Penitentiary at Terre Haute, Indiana, which is also discussed at length by the Presidential Commission (Mahoney et al. 1946). As the investigators describe it, the research 'was undertaken to evolve an infecting technique capable of consistently producing gonorrhoea in exposed populations' which could then be used to test prophylactic routines under clinical conditions. This was seen as superior to the alternative of simply treating disease in populations (like the military) with wide exposure. One of the qualifications to be a "volunteer" was 'assurance that the volunteer possessed a thorough understanding of the purpose underlying the study and the possible risks involved.' A 'financial reward' and 'certificate of participation' were provided, along with a 'suitable notation' in their prison record. More than 50 different ways to infect prisoners with gonorrhoea were tried. While no actual scrapping of the penis is described, the methods of attempting to produce disease were similar. In the initial experiment, 'The inoculum was retained in the urethra for five minutes through digital pressure at the meatus. During the interval, the glans and shaft of the penis were subjected to gentle massage and stretching. At the completion of the exposure the inoculum was allowed to escape, but urination was not permitted for one hour' (Mahoney et al. 1946).

Different levels of virulence in strains and amounts were used until clinical gonorrhoea was produced. The doses used were thought to be much higher than what might be acquired through normal intercourse, so more experiments were done to try to produce infection with lower exposures (and without massage) to find 'an adequate infecting routine.' Multiple strains were inoculated in multiple ways, but none 'proved capable of producing disease with a consistency considered to be adequate for a study of experimental prophylaxis' (Mahoney et al. 1946). All 'patients' who developed disease were treated with penicillin and cured. It is not much of a stretch to conclude that this set of experiments inspired the Guatemala prison experiments on syphilis—especially the search for a consistent method to produce venereal disease in humans. And it was to syphilis that Cutler turned after coming back to the US from Guatemala.

Cutler's syphilis studies were conducted at New York's Sing Sing prison, on 62 'human volunteers,' all males, at least 21 years old, more than two-thirds of whom were black, again with the goal of finding a reliable way to infect humans with disease (Magnuson et al. 1956). Fifty-four had some history of syphilis that had been treated in the past (they were grouped into five subgroups), and eight were 'non-syphilitic volunteers.' The authors of the Sing Sing research noted (correctly) that intentional infection with disease is only ethical because 'penicillin provides a safe and effective therapy for the disease.' Prisoners were recruited to the study primarily by a prison physician whom they trusted. The response was described as 'better than anticipated, although [unlike the Terra Haute experiments] no promise of money or special consideration was possible.' The main incentive was the guarantee that the prisoners would not be transferred from Sing Sing (described as 'one of the more desirable prisons in New York') until the completion of the study. 'This promise proved a potent one in soliciting volunteers.' The 'reasons for the study, the objectives, and the details of its day-to-day conduct' were discussed with potential volunteers (Magnuson et al. 1956).

The article summarises most of the syphilis research literature, noting that until the discovery of *T. pallidum* as the cause of syphilis in 1905, and the introduction of a rabbit model, direct inoculation of subjects was used 'in attempts to elucidate the nature of the disease.' Thereafter, 'the deliberate inoculation of nonsyphilitic humans ceased' and did not begin again, according to the authors, until it was shown that penicillin provided a 'safe and effective therapy for the disease' (Magnuson et al. 1956). Inoculations of both non-infectious killed antigen and the highly virulent strain of *T. pallidum* were injected into the prisoners' forearm. The study showed that it was possible to consistently produce disease in healthy prisoners, although (as before) the dose used was much higher than anyone would get through intercourse. It also demonstrated that persons with previously treated disease had a different response to a new infection (they are 'immunologically never the same'), though they could not be considered immune from re-infection. The authors concluded that most of their findings 'could be predicted by the animal [rabbit] data.' Nonetheless, in sentences that echo the then on-going Tuskegee study, they write: 'A few differences were observed. Experiments in the rabbits had not predicted the possible decline in immunity with the passage of time ... [but this could be simply related] to the relatively short life span of the experimental animal ... No animals have been followed for a 15–20 year period ... ' (Magnuson et al. 1956). The term "human volunteers" is used in the article's title, and sometimes in the article itself, but the term most frequently and consistently used to describe the prisoners in the study is "patients," as in, 'The patients were bled at bi-weekly intervals' (Magnuson et al. 1956).

These were both prison studies, as were most of the 41 direct-infection studies listed by NIH. Two nonprison studies in the list, nonetheless, are the most widely known, and are both much more ethically problematic than the Guatemala studies: the Jewish Chronic Disease Hospital and the Willowbrook experiments. The first involved the 1963 attempt to transplant cancer cells into 22 dying patients at the Jewish Chronic Disease Hospital in New York, chronicled in detail in Jay Katz's 1972 book, and also cited in the Beecher review (Langer 1966). The principal investigator of this study, Chester Southam, described the injection of live cancer cells into severely debilitated patients (he had previously done a similar study in 300 healthy prisoners) without their consent as 'routine medical practice.' In a 1964 affidavit, for example, Southam justified not telling the research subjects that they were being injected with 'cancer cells' on the basis that this was to protect their welfare as patients: 'I believe that such revelation is generally contraindicated in the best consideration of the patient's welfare and therefore to withhold such emotionally disturbing but medically nonpertinent details (unless requested by the patient) is in the best tradition of responsible clinical practice' (Katz 1972). As in Cutler's article, but even more directly, research is equated with treatment, subjects are viewed as patients, and researchers are transformed into treating physicians.

These self-deceptions are also inherent in doing research in disaster settings: disaster victims are viewed as patients needing treatment, researchers are seen (and see themselves) as treatment providers, and consent is ignored or marginalised because the immediate goal is to "help the victims," i.e. this is a humanitarian treatment mission. Of course, these observations apply only to disaster research in which consent is not or cannot be obtained. There may be minimal risk or no risk research in which consent in disaster settings is possible, and in which researchers see themselves as doing research, not humanitarian rescue work.

The other study that makes all three lists has become known as the Willowbrook study, in which hepatitis virus was fed to residents of a state home for the "mentally defective" to determine the protective effect of gamma globulin. 'The study group would include only patients whose parents gave consent' (Ward et al. 1958). Of a group of 16 residents, described as "patients," eleven were given gamma globulin prior to being fed double the 50 % infectivity dose of hepatitis virus, and five were fed the virus alone. Four of those five developed disease. Five months later the subjects were tested for immunity by being given the same viral dose. The results were inconclusive, so a follow-up study was done in which 16 "patients" were admitted directly to an isolation unit; ten were fed virus, and six were in "intimate contact" with them to serve as "controls." Four of the six controls developed hepatitis, suggesting that they acquired it from those who were fed the virus directly. All research subjects were consistently described as "patients" (Ward et al. 1958).

The Tuskegee study, which led Susan Reverby to discover the Guatemala study, is not on any of these lists, but is much better known than any of the other studies mentioned. Reverby's main point about Tuskegee, in contrast to Guatemala, is that no Tuskegee subjects were purposely infected by the researchers. While this is true, a more fundamental similarity between the Guatemala studies and Tuskegee is the total lack of informed consent of the research subjects, a lack not even mirrored in the pre-Nuremberg Code prison studies conducted in the US by Cutler. Cutler wrote his own 22-year update of the Tuskegee study in 1955, shortly after his Sing Sing study (Peters et al. 1955). At least two additional points are of note. First, in the "Untreated Syphilis in the Male Negro" article, Cutler and his colleagues continue the study's view that blacks experience syphilis differently than whites, even though Cutler himself had abandoned this view in his own research at Sing Sing; and second, remarkably, but consistent with his prison studies, the research subjects (who were consistently denied treatment for syphilis) are described in the article as "patients" (Peters et al. 1955).

We always act "shocked" by research scandals, often adopt new procedural mechanisms to try to prevent them in the future, but nonetheless usually see them as historical anomalies that cannot be repeated. We have, so far, always been wrong. Two disaster-related examples from the 1990s, a period not dealt with by Francis Collins (or anyone else) in responding to the Guatemala expose, explain why the Guatemala experiments are so threatening to contemporary researchers: the 076 studies and the Pfizer meningitis study. The first, the 076 maternal to child HIV/AIDS study, was, like the Guatemala experiments, sponsored by the US government in a developing country. It was justified as being a reasonable response to a disaster: the HIV/AIDS pandemic in Africa (Varmus 1997). It was criticised for applying an ethical double standard by using a placebo instead of a standard medical treatment in the control group, as well as for looking a lot like Tuskegee (Laurie 1997). Like Guatemala, it occasioned a joint response from the Centers for Disease Control and Prevention (CDC) and the NIH (the study's sponsors), who, among other things, denied the Tuskegee analogy, and argued that local standards (i.e., no care) rather than universal ones should be applied to the control group because it made the study more efficient so that an answer benefiting everyone in Africa could be arrived at faster (Varmus 1997). The proper question was (and remains) not what medical care was available to the African subjects, but what ethical obligations researchers owe to their subjects in terms of both rights and welfare. If, for example, the goal was to find a cheaper treatment, then the study was an economic one—requiring a demonstration that a cheaper treatment would actually be made available to the population (otherwise there would be no societal benefit) (Glantz et al. 1998).

The other example is the infamous Pfizer-sponsored meningitis study of the effectiveness of the new antibiotic Trovan on children in Nigeria during a meningitis epidemic (another "disaster") in 1997 (Annas 2009). Pfizer continues to publicly deny any wrongdoing, and even after agreeing to settle the lawsuits brought by parents for failure of obtain informed consent, pressured the Nigerian government to try to get the settlement terms lowered. A 2009 confidential cable from the US embassy in Nigeria, made public by WikiLeaks, quoted a Pfizer official as saying that the lawsuit against Pfizer had had a 'chilling effect' on international pharmaceutical companies who 'are no longer willing to conduct clinical testing in Nigeria. Liggeri [Enrico Liggeri, Pfizer Nigeria Country Director] opined that when another outbreak occurs no company will come to Nigeria's aid' (WikiLeaks Cables 2010). This is a remarkable statement, not least because Pfizer did not come to Nigeria's aid at all during their meningitis epidemic (there was no treatment involved, just experimentation), but used the epidemic opportunistically for its own goal of doing research using its drug Trovan, which it hoped to get FDA approval for use on children in the US (Annas 2009). Pfizer's actions also bred distrust of US-sponsored medical treatment in Nigeria, making it much more difficult to eradicate polio in the Kano area of the country. Neither the 076 study nor the Pfizer study were secret or justified as necessary for national security, but in both disaster studies it has been credibly alleged that informed consent was not obtained and that the subjects (or their parents) believed they were being treated for their illnesses, and were not involved in a clinical trial.

Guatemala is a "safe" subject for contemporary US researchers primarily because we have stopped using prisoners as research subjects (Hornblum 1988). Use of people institutionalised with mental disabilities, common in the 1940s and 1950s (Carter 1966), has also been discontinued. Intentionally infecting subjects with treatable diseases, most notably malaria, continues and remains accepted practice, although only with the informed consent of the subject and the availability of an effective treatment (Niiler 2010). What is different today, and what makes the Guatemala revelations potentially important, is that whereas in the immediate post-World War II era international research trials were the exception, today they have become the rule. One study, for example, concluded that in 2007 more than one-third of the trials sponsored by the 20 largest US-based pharmaceutical companies were being conducted outside of the US, and a majority of study sites were outside the US (Glickman 2009). The reason seems to be primarily financial, and ethical oversight is a 'major concern' (Glickman 2009). Studies on children are even more frequently done abroad, with one study finding that 65 % of published paediatric trials conducted from 1998 to 2007 included sites outside the US, involving 54 countries (Pasquali et al. 2010). The FDA has not been able to keep pace, inspecting fewer than 1 % of foreign clinical trial sites (Office of Inspector General 2010). Of course some of these trials are conducted in countries with reasonable research oversight, but the majority are conducted in countries where research oversight is problematic at best.

This is why Guatemala "horrifies" us. We want to believe, with the Presidential Commission, that it can't happen again, but we know it can. Globalised research today is not done in secret like a CIA or military operation (at least not outside of the "black sites," Guantanamo, and Abu Ghraib), at least not by private corporations and academic researchers. Nonetheless, we simply don't know what's going on around the world in regard to research on humans (Pasquali 2010; Office of Inspector General 2010). We have mostly taken research out of the prisons and mental institutions, but have substituted poor people in developing countries as "go to" subjects, and outsourced oversight to the private sector of contract research organizations and pharmaceutical companies (Petryna 2009; Petryna et al. 2006). IRBs are now for hire and informed consent has been transformed from a process to a paper form, the drafting of which is an exercise between the investigators and the members of IRBs. In this context, current proposals are not to strengthen the informed consent process, but to reduce the paperwork by making the consent forms shorter (Emanuel and Menikoff 2011). This is not surprising if researchers see consent as mechanical book-keeping that is meaningless to research subjects (patients, victims) and just a hoop they have to jump through to do their important research and reassure their compliance officers. Informed consent forms in the immediate aftermath of a disaster have about as much relevance (arguably even less) to the protection of the rights of the victim-subjects as would giving them a Barney-the-purple-dinosaur doll.

9.4 Conclusion

Globalisation of research trials is the new reality, and it provides a new context for two old and as yet unmet challenges: transparency, and meaningful informed consent. As Jay Katz noted, as a member of both the Tuskegee review panel and the Human Radiation Experiments panel, although informed consent is central to protecting the rights and welfare of research subjects, we have consistently 'failed to take responsibility for making . . . informed consent meaningful' (Advisory Committee 1966). This is the lesson and continuing challenge of Nuremberg, Guatemala, Tuskegee, the Human Radiation Experiments, the military and CIA experiments, and US globalised research generally. And this is the context in which a new category of research, "disaster research," has been suggested. We should give special attention to disaster victims, and it is reasonable to discuss what kinds of research might be appropriate to perform on them. But this discussion should not (and thankfully outside of the military and CIA generally has not) include proposals to abolish or marginalize informed consent. There is no exception in international law for informed consent in disasters, and there should not be. It is, I think, critical that researchers who propose doing "disaster research," and IRBs who review their proposals, not even attempt to have this area of research become an exception to the ethical and legal requirement for informed consent (London 2009). Human beings don't lose their human rights by having a heart attack or by being the victims of a natural disaster or a war. Moreover, it is easy to confuse the rescuer-victim relationship with the doctor-patient relationship, especially when the rescue involves medical treatment.

Nor can anticipatory IRB review of disaster research proposals before an actual disaster happens protect subjects. Paul Farmer explains why in reflecting on disasters a year after the Haiti earthquake; all disasters are unique:

> Since January 12 (2010) countries as different as Japan, Cuba, Mexico, and Brazil offered pragmatic assistance to Haiti by drawing on their own experiences with disasters. Some of this assistance proved helpful. But the circumstances in Japan and China and Brazil—even neighboring Cuba—seemed so different from those in Haiti. Even when the acute insult—an earthquake or a hurricane—was the same, the chronic malady was very different. (Farmer 2011)

We make a similar mistake in our "all-hazards preparedness" doctrine: preparing for an earthquake does not help us prepare for a biological or chemical attack, or even for a flu pandemic (Annas 2010). All disasters really are unique. Disasters can also be opportunities. Disasters are opportunities to help the victims, they should not be used as opportunities to exploit victims by doing research on them without their consent. Informed consent is not a purple dinosaur that can or should be displaced in disasters by good intentions: it is the sine qua non of protecting human dignity and promoting human rights (Annas 2010).

More important than novel research proposals, reflection on medical research ethics in disasters provides an opportunity to re-examine the linkage between human rights and bioethics, a linkage embodied in UNESCO's Universal Declaration on Bioethics and Human Rights. Such a framework requires the informed consent of research subjects, but as important, requires a social justice perspective of global benefit sharing through 'macrolevel distribution of basic goods and opportunities' (Solbakk 2011). Research on victims' health and healthcare needs cannot reasonably be conducted in the immediate aftermath of a disaster, when all resources should go to rescue. But the attention span of the international "first responders" is very short (Farmer 2011).

After the immediate care in a disaster has been given, when the first responders have left, and when attention can be turned to rebuilding infrastructure and restoring health, conducting research on human survivors may become more reasonable (Collogan et al. 2004). It is, for example, unreasonable to do a randomised clinical trial of limb amputations in the immediate aftermath of an earthquake. It is, however, perfectly reasonable to do a follow-up study to see how those who had amputations fared as compared to those who refused to consent to amputation. Research in the rebuilding stage of a disaster aftermath may also serve to retain at least some international interest in the lives and health of the disaster survivors. Humans have generally reacted well in disasters by trying to help our fellow humans in danger. The challenge is to make temporary, disaster-driven, identification with the impoverished and endangered peoples of the world permanent, and to work to maximise global human dignity and health in everyday life.

References

Advisory Committee on Human Radiation Experiments. 1996. *The Human Radiation Experiments: Final Report of the President's Advisory Committee*. New York: Oxford University Press.

Annas, George J. 1998. Protecting soldiers from friendly fire: The consent requirement for using investigational drugs and vaccines in combat. *American Journal of Law & Medicine* 24: 245–260.

Annas, George J. 2009. Globalized clinical trials and informed consent. *New England Journal of Medicine* 360: 2050–2053.

Annas, George J. 2010. *Worst case bioethics: Death, destruction, and public health*. New York: Oxford University Press.

Annas, George J., and Michael A. Grodin. 1992. *The Nazi doctors and the Nuremberg code: Human rights in human experimentation*. New York: Oxford University Press.

Beecher, Henry K. 1966. Ethics and clinical research. *New England Journal of Medicine* 274: 1354–1360.

Carter, Richard. 1966. *Breakthrough: The saga of Jonas Salk*. New York: Trident Press.

Collogan, Lauren K., Farris Tuma, Regina Dolan-Sewell, Susan Borja, and Alan R. Fleischman. 2004. Ethical issues pertaining to research in the aftermath of disaster. *Journal of Traumatic Stress* 17: 363–372.

Emanuel, Ezekiel J., and Jerry Menikoff. 2011. Reforming the regulations governing research with human subjects. *New England Journal of Medicine* 365: 1145–1150.

Farmer, Paul. 2011. *Haiti after the earthquake*. New York: Public Affairs.

Fost, Norman. 1998. Waived consent for emergency research. American Journal of Law and. *Medicine* 24:163–183.

Fox News.com. 2010. US government apologizes for 1940s STD testing on Guatemalans. Oct 1, 2010. http://www.foxnews.com/politics/2010/10/01/government-apologizes-s-std-testing-guatemalans/. Accessed 21 October 2011.

Frieden, Thomas R., and Francis S. Collins. 2010. Intentional infection of vulnerable populations in 1946–1948: Another tragic history lesson. *Journal of the American Medical Association* 304: 2063–2064.

Funes, Juan M., John C. Cutler, Sacha Levitan, Jay Portnoy, and Rolando Funes. 1953. Estudios serologicos y clinicos con referencia a la sifilis en Guatemala, Centro America: II. Observaciones efectuadas en un grupo de ninos de escuela en el Puerto de San Jose. *Boletin de la Oficina Sanitaria Panamericana* 34: 14–18.

Glantz, Leonard H., George J. Annas, Michael A. Grodin, and Wendy K. Mariner. 1998. Research in developing countries: taking 'benefit' seriously. *Hastings Center Report no* 6:38–42.

Glickman, Seth W., John G. McHutchison, Eric D. Peterson, Charles B. Cairns, Robert A. Harrington, Robert M. Califf, and Kevin A. Schulman. 2009. Ethical and scientific implications of the globalization of clinical research. *New England Journal of Medicine* 360: 816–823.

Graniger, Sarah., and Carol Rosenberg. 2010. U.S. apologizes to Guatemalans for 1940s STD experiment. Miami Herald, A1, October 1.

Guidance for Institutional Review Boards. 2011. Clinical Investigators, and Sponsors. Exception from Informed Consent Requirements for Emergency Research, HHS. http://www.fda.gov/downloads/RegulatoryInformation/Guidances/UCM249673.pdf. Accessed 21 October 2011.

Hornblum, Allen M. 1998. *Acres of skin: Human experiments at Holmesburg Prison*. New York: Routledge.

Jones, James. 1981. *Bad blood: the Tuskegee syphilis experiment*. New York: Free Press.

Katz, Jay. 1972. *Experimentation with human beings*. New York: Russell Sage Foundation.

Langer, Elinor. 1966. Human experimentation: New York verdict affirms patient's rights. *Science* 151: 665–666.

London, Alex John. 2009. Clinical research in a public health crisis: the integrative approach to managing uncertainty and mitigating conflict. *Seton Hall Law Review* 39: 1173–1202.

Lurie, Peter., and Sidney M. Wolfe. 1997. Unethical trials of interventions to reduce perinatal transmission of the human immunodeficiency virus in developing countries. *New England Journal of Medicine* 337: 853–856.

Magnuson, Harold J., Evan W. Thomas, Sidney Olansky, Bernard L. Kaplan, Lopo de Mello, and John C. Cutler. 1956. Inoculation syphilis in human volunteers. *Medicine* 35: 33–82.

Mahoney, John F., Cassius James Van Slyke, John C. Cutler, and Henrik L. Blum. 1946. Experimental gonococcic urethritis in human volunteers. *American Journal of Syphilis, Gonorrhea, and Venereal Disease* 30:1–39.

McNeil, Donald G. 2010. U.S. Apologizes for syphilis tests in Guatemala, New York Times, October 1. http://www.nytimes.com/2010/10/02/health/research/02infect.html. Accessed 21 October 2011.

Niiler, Eric. 2010. Volunteers at Walter Reed endure mosquito bites to help find a malaria vaccine. Washington Post, HE01, September 7. http://www.washingtonpost.com/wp-dyn/content/article/2010/09/03/AR2010090305111.html?sub=AR. Accessed 21 October 2011.

Office of Inspector General, Department Health and Human Services. 2010. Challenges to FDA's ability to monitor and inspect foreign clinical trials (OPEI-01-08-00510). http://oig.hhs.gov/oei/reports/oei-01–08-00510.pdf. Accessed 21 October 2011.

Pasquali Sara, K., S. Burstein Danielle, K. Benjamin Daniel, Smith Brian, Jennifer S. Li and. 2010. Globalization of pediatric research: Analysis of clinical trials completed for pediatric exclusivity. *Pediatrics* 126: e687–692.

Peters, John J., Peers JH, Sidney Olansky, John C. Cutler, and Geraldine A. Gleeson. 1955. Untreated syphilis in the male negro. *Journal of Chronic Disease* 1: 127–148.

Petryna, Adriana., Andrew Lakoff, and Arthur Kleinman, eds. 2006. *Global pharmaceuticals: Ethics, markets, practices*. Durham: Duke University Press.

Petryna, Adriana. 2009. *When experiments travel: Clinical trials and the global search for human subjects*. Princeton: Princeton University Press.

Presidential Commission for the Study of Bioethical Issues. 2011. "Ethically Impossible": STD Research in Guatemala from 1946 to 1948. http://www.bioethics.gov/cms/sites/default/files/Ethically-Impossible_PCSBI.pdf. Accessed 21 October 2011.

Reverby, Susan M., ed. 2000. *Tuskegee's truths: Rethinking the Tuskegee syphilis study*. Chapel Hill: University of North Carolina Press.

Reverby, Susan M. 2009. *Examining Tuskegee: The infamous syphilis study and its legacy*. Chapel Hill: University of North Carolina Press.

Reverby, Susan M. 2011. "Normal exposure" and inoculation syphilis: A PHS "Tuskegee" doctor in Guatemala, 1946–1948. *Journal of Policy History* 23: 6–24.

Ronson, Jon. 2004. *The men who stare at goats*. New York: Simon and Schuster Paperbacks.

Shuster, Evelyne 2013. Chapter 8, this volume.

Smith, Stephen. 2010. Wellesley professor unearths a horror: syphilis experiments in Guatemala, US apologizes for performing unethical study in the 1940s. Boston Globe, B1, October 2. http://www.boston.com/news/local/massachusetts/articles/2010/10/02/wellesley_professor_unearths_a_horror_syphilis_experiments_in_guatemala/. Accessed 21 October 2011.

Solbakk, Jan Helge. 2011. In the ruins of Babel: pitfalls on the way toward a universal language for research ethics and benefit sharing. *Cambridge Quarterly of Healthcare Ethics* 20: 1–15.

Stein, Rob. 2010. U.S. infected Guatemalans for STD tests, Washington Post, A1, October 2. http://www.washingtonpost.com/wp-dyn/content/article/2010/10/01/AR2010100107299.html. Accessed 21 October 2011.

Stout, Genevieve W., and, John C. Cutler. 1951. Serology problems (syphilis) in Central America. *Journal of Venereal Disease Information* 32: 237–241.

Transcript, US Department of State. 2010. Briefing on the U.S. Public Health Services STD Inoculation Study of 1946–1948 Via Teleconference. October 1. http://www.state.gov/p/wha/rls/rm/2010/148546.htm. Accessed 21 October 2011.

U.S. v. Stanley, 483 U.S. 669 (1987).

Varmus, Harold., and David Satcher. 1997. Ethical complexities of conducting research in developing countries. *New England Journal of Medicine* 337: 1003–1005.

Ward, Robert., Saul Krugman, Joan P. Giles, A. Milton Jacobs, and Oscar Bodansky. 1958. Infectious hepatitis: Studies of its natural history and prevention. *New England Journal of Medicine* 258: 407–416.

Weiner, Tim. 2007. *Legacy of ashes: The history of the CIA*. New York: Doubleday.

WikiLeaks. 2010. Boseley, Sarah., WikiLeaks cables: Pfizer 'used dirty tricks to avoid clinical trial payout', Guardian, Dec 9, 2010 [US embassy cables: Pfizer nears $75 m Nigeria settlement, cable text released by WikiLeaks and published by the Guardian. http://www.guardian.co.uk/business/2010/dec/09/wikileaks-cables-pfizer-nigeria. Accessed 21 October 2011.

Chapter 10
Setting Disaster Research Priorities

Virginia Murray and Anthony Kessel

10.1 Introduction

Disaster research priorities are complex and difficult to set, but are vital for the rapid advancement of the scientific evidence base for disaster risk reduction and planning, and for enabling better response to humanitarian and health catastrophes. To some degree, the processes to identify disaster research priorities will depend on systems within countries, regions and international organisations. Some of these might be specific to the disaster context while others are used more generally in research prioritisation. Yet there has been very little written to our knowledge, in any language, on setting disaster research priorities let alone examining the ethical issues pertaining to such priority setting.

The chapter will be organised around three broad existing approaches to setting disaster research priorities. We will explore each one critically, examining its advantages and disadvantages. The ethical aspects raised by each approach will be addressed.

10.2 Approach A: Healthcare Priority Setting

To enhance the decision making process around setting research priorities in a disaster context, it may be helpful to consider the principles around priority setting that have been developed in relation to healthcare resources. Over the past two decades an extensive literature on priority setting within healthcare has developed as issues of 'rationing' or 'resource allocation' have become more prominent (Anand et al. 2004). It is important to note, however, that most of this literature has related to priority setting around health care services or health technologies, rather than around setting

V. Murray (✉) · A. Kessel
Public Health England, London, UK
e-mail: Virginia.Murray@phe.gov.uk

D. P. O'Mathúna et al. (eds.), *Disaster Bioethics: Normative Issues When Nothing is Normal,* Public Health Ethics Analysis 2, DOI 10.1007/978-94-007-3864-5_10,

priorities for public health programmes or indeed for research, let alone for disaster research. The academic health literature has also tended to focus on theoretical aspects of priority setting. There is relatively little in terms of practical guides or decision making tools, especially for public health organisations or public health policy makers (Rhodes et al. 2002).

Daniels and Sabin have argued persuasively for several years that, although it has not been possible to gain consensus on the exact principles (or criteria) that should determine the setting of priorities, there is good agreement on the nature of the process (Daniels and Sabin 2008).

An approach put forward by Daniels is called 'accountability for reasonableness', and describes the need for a fair, deliberative process to establish the legitimacy and fairness of priority setting decisions (Daniels 2000). He asserts the importance of holding decision makers accountable for the reasonableness of their decisions, and stresses the importance of meeting the following elements, discussed in more detail later.

a. transparency—the process must be public (fully transparent) about the grounds for its decisions;
b. relevance—decisions must rest on reasons that stakeholders can agree are relevant;
c. revisability—decisions should be revisable in light of new evidence and arguments; and
d. assurance—there should be assurance through enforcement that these conditions (transparency, relevance, and revisability) will be upheld.

Further work suggests that the form that procedures should take depends on the institutional context (Gruskin and Daniels 2008). In addition, decisions are constrained by more general considerations of justice, such as the requirement that they not be discriminatory. Other authors have stressed the parallel importance of human rights (Gruskin and Daniels 2008).

Underlying these points is the importance of having an understanding of social value judgements. By drawing on experience from priority setting in the National Health Service (NHS) in the UK, the National Institute for Health and Clinical Excellence (NICE) published guidance on social value judgements (NICE 2008), which may be helpful for setting disaster research priorities. In summary, the social value judgements expounded by NICE are:

i) moral principles,
ii) procedural justice,
iii) fundamental operating principles,
iv) evidence-based decision-making,
v) avoiding discrimination and promoting equality.

These concepts will be discussed briefly in turn below.

10.2.1 Moral Principles

These are concepts that include:

- respect for autonomy (allowing individual choices without undue influence). Influence is a complex concept within ethics. For example, undue influence can be described as occurring through offers of excessive, unwarranted, inappropriate or improper reward or other overtures in order to obtain compliance (NCPHSBBR 1979);
- non-maleficence (most simply explained as 'First, do no harm');
- beneficence (active goodness); and
- social (distributive) justice—distributive justice is a concept that is concerned with the fair allocation of resources among diverse members of a community. The issue of fair allocation is typically that which takes into account the total amount of goods to be distributed, the distributing procedure, and the pattern of distribution that results (Maiese, 2003).

10.2.2 Procedural Justice

This addresses the concept of 'accountability for reasonableness.' Daniels and Sabin (1997) have described the conditions that make up their concept of accountability for reasonableness, as mentioned previously:

- Transparency—limit-setting decisions and their rationales must be publicly accessible.
- Relevance—the rationale must rest on information and principled arguments that fair-minded parties (people predisposed to working together under rules of mutual cooperation) can agree are relevant to deciding how to meet the diverse needs of a covered population under necessary resource constraints.
- Appeals—there is a mechanism for challenge and dispute resolution regarding limit-setting decisions, including the opportunity for revising decisions in light of further evidence or arguments.
- Enforcement—there is either voluntary or public regulation of the process to ensure that the first three conditions are met.

However, Gibson and colleagues (2002)considered that a limitation of 'accountability for reasonableness' was that it did not sufficiently explain how an institution could operationalise the concept. NICE have considered this and they describe procedural justice as including publicity, relevance, challenge and revision as well as regulation.

10.2.3 Operating Principles

Fundamental operating principles are more straightforward and include legal obligations and procedural principles covering scientific rigour, inclusiveness, transparency, independence, challenge, review, support for implementation and timeliness.

10.2.4 Evidence-based Decision-making

This approach is familiar to health professionals and professionals in other settings. This concept covers clinical and public health effectiveness and cost effectiveness. Of note such decision-making includes comparing the cost effectiveness of different interventions in relation to:

- individual choice (in other words the right to choose);
- rare conditions—for example rare diseases requiring ultra-orphan drugs to treat exceptionally low patient numbers are difficult to assess by an evidence base (Hughes et al. 2005). Ultra-orphan drugs are expensive to produce for pharmaceutical companies who find it difficult to recoup research and development costs, so are invariably cost-ineffective. These drugs provide an example of how evidence-based decision-making is complex and can lead to issues associated with the pleading of 'special cases' which may not be regarded as equitable for the wider community.
- the 'rule of rescue'—this has been described as 'the imperative people feel to rescue identifiable individuals facing avoidable death' (McKie and Richardson 2003).

10.2.5 Avoiding Discrimination and Promoting Equality

The final social value judgment includes issues relating to race, disability, age, sex/gender, sexual orientation, religion, beliefs and socioeconomic status. All of these point towards the importance of reducing health inequalities.

These healthcare based principles for setting priorities are valuable and reflect wider issues pertaining to healthcare ethics and human rights. Box 9.1 provides two examples of how the NICE social value judgements have been used in practice:

Box 10.1. NICE social value judgements used in practice

- NICE assessed the use of a drug called capecitabine for the treatment of inoperable advanced gastric cancer. In their summary on the social value judgements they reported that 'the Committee considered whether there were issues related to equality to be taken into account in its considerations' (NICE 2010, p. 13). The report went on to state that 'it acknowledged that some people with inoperable advanced gastric cancer may not be able to swallow oral capecitabine tablets because of difficulty with swallowing as a result of the cancer, or because of nausea' (NICE 2010, p. 13). In conclusion the committee considered that 'there were no specific issues relating to equality that needed to be taken into account' (NICE 2010, p. 17).

- NICE have considered the use of the drug mifamurtide in combination with postoperative multi-agent chemotherapy as an option for the treatment of high-grade resectable non-metastatic osteosarcoma after macroscopically complete surgical resection in children, adolescents and young adults, and when mifamurtide is made available at a reduced cost to the NHS under the patient access scheme. In the equalities considerations and social value judgements of the committee's assessment they stated that the 'comments made at the scoping stage relating to equalities issues included the observation that osteosarcoma mainly affects children, teenagers and young adults, and that osteosarcoma is a rare disease'(NICE 2010, p. 33). Further 'the Committee was therefore satisfied that there were no equalities issues relating to age in this appraisal and that the recommendations were consistent with NICE's obligations under the equalities legislation and the requirement for fairness' (NICE 2010, p. 33).

The principles and approaches outlined in this section for setting priorities in healthcare appear to be relevant to the context of setting disaster research priorities for two related reasons. First, those who are the victims of disasters have heightened need of healthcare services, so having principles to inform such access would appear useful. Second, the importance of better understanding of health and health service needs during disasters is paramount, and so such principles can help guide acquisition of new research knowledge to enhance the evidence base.

10.3 Approach B: Organisations that have Set Disaster Research Priorities

Another way of exploring the setting of disaster research priorities is to look at organisations that have already attempted to set such priorities, and to examine the processes they used. In this section we investigate four organisations, selected because they are among the few to have published disaster research priorities and because they represent a range of organisational types:

- Médecins Sans Frontières (MSF)—an internationally recognised and operating non-governmental organisation (NGO);

- Enhanced Learning and Research for Humanitarian Assistance (EHLRA)—a UK collaborative development between academia and humanitarian partners;
- International Council for Science (ICSU) and its Integrated Research on Disaster Risk (IRDR); and
- Health Protection Agency (HPA)—a national public health body in the UK.

10.3.1 Médecins Sans Frontières

Médecins Sans Frontières (MSF) is an internationally, highly regarded NGO that has worked as an independent medical humanitarian organisation in over 70 countries. It has provided medical assistance for over 35 years to populations vulnerable through conflict, disease and inadequate health systems.

In 2005, MSF published their Ethics Framework for Medical Research, which considered the ethical principles pertaining to international research including collaborative partnerships, social value, scientific validity, fair selection of study population, favourable harm-benefit ratio, informed consent, respect for recruited participants and study communities, and independent review (MSF 2005).

In an article on ethical dilemmas in medical humanitarian practice, Sheather and Shah (2011) presented ethics case studies for field staff, and training modules on medical ethics for managers and doctors. For this purpose they used three case studies on HIV testing, on female genital mutilation and on acting beyond competence. Each case study described the problem, the MSF dilemma, the ethicist's response and the outcome for the relevant MSF programme. The authors concluded by stating that by 'working with communities, by raising awareness of the benefits that medicine can bring, so attitudes change' and that intractable dilemmas today might be 'forgotten tomorrow' (Sheather and Shah 2011, p. 165). Their aim was to invite open discussion and dialogue in the wider medical community working in crisis, conflict or with severe resource limitations.

The principles laid out by MSF (2005) combine ethical issues around health research with ethical issues connected to resource allocation, which together provide a helpful guide to setting disaster research priorities—and are complementary to the principles described by Sheather and Shah (2011). They state that medical ethics defines the starting point of the relationship between medical staff and patients. They report that the MSF charter and guiding documents state that 'MSF volunteers undertake to respect their professional code of ethics' and that 'MSF missions are carried out in the respect of the rules of medical ethics, in particular the duty to provide care without causing harm to either individuals or groups. Each person in danger will be assisted with humanity, impartiality and in respect of medical confidentiality' (Sheather and Shah 2011, p. 162).

10.3.2 Enhanced Learning and Research for Humanitarian Assistance

Launched in 2009, Enhanced Learning and Research for Humanitarian Assistance (ELRHA) presents its vision for a global humanitarian community where humanitarian actors actively collaborate with higher education institutes to noticeably reduce risk and to ensure that those suffering from the impact of disasters receive more timely, relevant and sustainable assistance (ELRHA 2011a). ELHRA aims to develop highly professional responders, to share expertise and to carry out research.

ELHRA is funded by the UK Department for Employment and Learning, the Higher Education Funding Council for England, the Higher Education Funding Council for Wales, and the Scottish Further and Higher Education Funding Council, and is hosted by Save the Children. To link to the broader international agenda, ELHRA has a particular focus on building collaborative partnerships with universities in the UK, where the wealth of academic expertise and the presence of some of the world's leading humanitarian agencies combine to create a unique environment with the potential to provide a world leading centre for humanitarian research and training.

ELHRA has four thematic underpinnings to its research priority areas, which are collaborative working, innovation and future preparedness, humanitarian principles and operational challenges. Accountability is used to describe ELRHA's main ethical thrust for ensuring the importance of the people, attitudes and behaviours of humanitarian staff and they are concerned to ensure that relief is accountable (ELRHA 2011b).

ELHRA is currently one of the few innovations that the authors are aware of where academia and humanitarian assistance meet to enhance each other's work, and provides another framework within which to consider the setting of disaster research priorities.

10.3.3 International Council for Science

The International Council for Science (ICSU) is an NGO with a global membership of national scientific bodies (121 members, representing 141 countries) and International Scientific Unions (30 members). ICSU's mission is to strengthen international science for the benefit of society by mobilising the knowledge and resources of the international science community to:

> Identify and address major issues of importance to science and society; facilitate interaction amongst scientists across all disciplines and from all countries; promote participation of all scientists—regardless of race, citizenship, language, political stance, or gender— in the international scientific endeavour; and to provide independent, authoritative advice to stimulate constructive dialogue between the scientific community and governments, civil society, and the private sector. (ICSU 2004, p. 1)

In 2004 the ICSU Foresight Analysis, which was developed for their own Committee on Scientific Planning and Review, stated that natural disasters pose a serious threat to populations around the world, each year causing thousands of lives lost, millions of people injured or displaced, and billions of dollars in damage (ICSU 2004). The analysis considered the different ways in which the scientific community may contribute to reducing society's vulnerability to such events, which can help prevent hazards from turning into disasters. From their report it is interesting to see the examples of critical scientific and technical challenges they identified, which provides a foundation for setting disaster research priorities: improving the ability to predict events such as droughts, floods, hurricanes, and landslides; strengthening understanding of the basic physics underlying earthquake generation through the integration of new observational tools, and developing engineering responses to reduce the impacts of seismic activity; and assessing the potential for increased vulnerability of particular regions to natural disasters as a result of anthropogenically-driven changes in climate and land use.

In 2005, the ICSU Priority Area Assessment report, *Capacity Building in Science*, stated that many of the most serious problems facing humanity in the 21st century are not limited by national boundaries (ICSU 2006). The report notes that poverty and ignorance are present in all countries, and that the threats of climate change, depletion of the oceans, the spread of HIV, and other pandemics and natural disasters are challenges to all of humanity.

Three years later a report, under ICSU's Integrated Research on Disaster Reduction (IRDR), was presented which proposed that a series of in-depth, post-disaster, multi-disciplinary investigations be carried out, with the primary objective of describing the limits of existing knowledge and identifying a set of key research questions (ICSU 2008).

In the most immediate period, ICSU's relevance to setting disaster research priorities has remained prominent. In a 2003 document, a Priority Area Assessment Panel report on *Environment and Its Relation to Sustainable Development*, ICSU identified the issue of hazards as a priority (ICSU 2003).

The Priority Area Assessment Panel concluded that there exists a great deal of knowledge and research excellence on issues such as the analysis and design of infrastructure and public health systems, severe weather, earthquakes and other hazardous events, and public policy questions on the management of risk and interactions among different levels of government. However, the report critiques the fact that much of the research is conducted along single-disciplinary lines, and has had a retrospective rather than futuristic view.

The Priority Area Assessment report recommended the creation of a new ICSU/IRDR led programme on 'Natural and Human-induced Hazards' that addresses critical infrastructure, population health, hazards assessment and international development with these priorities being set by the members of the Committee from their knowledge, experience and discussions. An integrated risk management approach would examine the intersection of vulnerabilities and hazards

10.3.4 Health Protection Agency

The Health Protection Agency (HPA) is an independent organisation that was set up by the UK government in 2003 to protect the public from threats to their health from infectious diseases and environmental hazards (HPA 2011a). It does this by providing advice and information to the general public, to health professionals such as doctors and nurses, and to national and local government. The functions of the Agency are set down in legislation and are described as protecting the community (or any part of the community) against infectious diseases and other dangers to health (UK Government 2004). Within HPA's research and development programme the aims and objectives for all research carried out by the HPA include complying with UK research governance guidelines and standards for best practice. In April 2013 the HPA merged with a number of other organisations to form Public Health England, where standards for setting research priorities are maintained.

The HPA has undertaken research gap analyses. For example in March 2009 a two-day workshop with over 80 participants addressed environmental exposure and health with the Medical Research Council (MRC), the Natural Environment Research Council and others (Weber and Culshaw 2009). One of the questions addressed was 'What are the key research gaps, needs and opportunities that the UK is particularly well placed to address?' In the meeting conclusions, opportunities were identified which included the need for a joint UK funding initiative to stimulate multi-disciplinary and integrated approaches related to the health and environmental sciences. This could bring in other areas, such as social sciences and engineering, to tackle real world problems using innovative methodologies, and support training and capacity building in quantitative skills across disciplines to build sustainable networks of excellence (Weber and Culshaw 2009).

As a result of this workshop a new MRC-HPA Centre for Environment & Health at Imperial College and King's College, London was created with sponsorship from the MRC, the Department of Health and HPA to build better evidence. This centre has a mission statement that states it will 'undertake the highest quality research in the fields of public health, in order to inform the policy and understanding of the key issues affecting society. The Centre will achieve this by bringing together the best researchers from all areas of public health, encouraging novel cross disciplinary approaches, and providing the highest quality training to new and existing researchers in these fields. The Centre is based upon the principles of openness, transparency, and integrity in all of our work, with the primary goal of improving national and international public health' (IC/KCL 2011). Areas of research undertaken by this MRC-HPA centre include health risk assessment, and extreme events and disaster management and response planning.

The HPA's targets are listed in its Strategic Overview 2010–2015 as reducing key infections, minimising the health impact of environmental hazards including radiation, chemicals and poisons, and supporting safe and effective biological medicines (HPA 2010). In this overview the need was formally stated to develop the evidence base for public health effects from extreme environmental events and climate change;

in part this was a consequence of the 2003 heat wave (Kovats et al. 2006), floods across England in 2007 (Pitt 2008) and volcanic ash over the UK in 2010 (Elliot et al. 2010). Concerns arising from these disasters led to the establishment of the Extreme Events and Health Protection Section (EEHPS) in 2011 (HPA 2011b). The section has an active research programme covering human health impacts from floods, heat, cold, volcanic ash, thunderstorm asthma and other disaster risk reduction resources.

In May 2011, via EEHPS, the HPA worked with WHO and UNISDR to make available *Disaster Risk Management for Health Fact Sheets* (WHO/HPA/UNISDR 2011). These fact sheets were prepared to develop capacities for health disaster risk management. These two-page advocacy sheets address the following topics: Chemical safety, Child health, Climate Change management, Communicable disease, Disabilities, Mass casualty management, Mass fatalities, Mental health and psychosocial support, Non-communicable diseases, Nutrition, Radiation emergencies, Safe hospitals, Sexual and reproductive health, and Water sanitation and hygiene. This work has led to HPA being designated as a WHO Collaborating Centre on Mass Gatherings and Extreme Events.

10.3.5 Comparing Disaster Research Priority-setting Strategies

The four organisations described above are all involved in setting disaster research priorities. Their knowledge and experience needs to be taken into account to ensure ethical issues are given appropriate consideration in future developments.

MSF undertakes front line response and some research, and is very much aware of the importance of ethical principles. Their achievements in this area are highly commendable. The ELHRA is a new body, working to support frontline humanitarian aid which is aware of the key role of accountability in promoting ethical practice. The ICSU and its IRDR likewise accept that there is an inescapable ethical dimension to disaster research. The HPA sets disaster research priorities and in many areas has Research Ethics Committees.

MSF has published its ethical principles pertaining to international research studies (MSF 2005; see Chap. 12). These principles include collaborative partnerships, social value, scientific validity, fair selection of study population, favourable harm-benefit ratio, informed consent, respect for recruited participants and study communities, and independent review. This approach is valuable and could be developed into a standard that other organisations conducting disaster research studies could benefit from. However, as far as this chapter's authors are aware, it is not apparent that these organisations have published the ethical principles they use in setting disaster research priorities.

10.4 Approach C: The Hyogo Framework for Action

The International Strategy for Disaster Reduction (ISDR) is a strategic framework, adopted by United Nations (UN) Member States in 2000, aiming to guide and coordinate the efforts of a wide range of partners to achieve substantive reduction in disaster losses and build resilient nations and communities (UNISDR 2011a).

The UNISDR serves as the focal point for the implementation of the *Hyogo Framework for Action 2005–2015: Building the Resilience of Nations and Communities to Disasters* (UNISDR 2007)—a plan of action adopted by 168 governments to protect lives and livelihoods against disasters. Three strategic goals were adopted within this framework: a) the more effective integration of disaster risk considerations into sustainable development policies, planning and programming at all levels, with a special emphasis on disaster prevention, mitigation, preparedness and vulnerability reduction; b) the development and strengthening of institutions, mechanisms and capacities at all levels, in particular at the community level, that can systematically contribute to building resilience to hazards; and c) the systematic incorporation of risk reduction approaches into the design and implementation of emergency preparedness, response and recovery programmes in the reconstruction of affected communities.

From these strategic goals under the Hyogo Framework for Action (HFA), the priorities are to:

- Ensure that disaster risk reduction is a national and a local priority with a strong institutional basis for implementation.
- Identify, assess and monitor disaster risks and enhance early warning.
- Use knowledge, innovation and education to build a culture of safety and resilience at all levels.
- Reduce the underlying risk factors.
- Strengthen disaster preparedness for effective response at all levels. (UNISDR 2007)

As a result of this and other activities, a UNISDR Science and Technical Committee was subsequently developed. In their 2009 report, *Reducing Disaster Risks through Science: Issues and Actions*, the committee recommends a greater emphasis on transferring knowledge into action, using a problem-solving approach that integrates all hazards and disciplines, supporting systematic science programmes, and guiding good practice in scientific and technical aspects of disaster risk reduction. The report suggests that the 'ISDR Scientific and Technical Committee should be strengthened to serve as a neutral, credible international resource to support practitioners at all levels, from local through national to international levels, by overseeing the collection, vetting and publicising of information on good practices carried out on the basis of sound science and up-to-date scientific and technological knowledge, as well as on those inadequate practices or concepts that may be hindering progress' (UNISDR 2009a, p. 5; UNISDR 2009b, p. viii). Currently this committee's remit has not yet been to set disaster research priorities, so it has not had to consider the related ethical issues.

The on-going work of the UNISDR Science and Technical Committee and partner agencies is allowing various activities to develop, including those of the Intergovernmental Panel on Climate Change (IPCC 2009) which led to a special report on *Managing the Risks of Extreme Events and Disasters to Advance Climate Change Adaptation* (IPCC 2012). This collaborative opportunity allows the research priorities of international UN based organisations to fit with the needs of local, national and other international organisations.

In the HFA Mid-Term Review, published in March 2011, it was reported that in the study commissioned on the use of databases for disaster risk reduction that 'much of the existing operational research related to emergencies and disasters lacks consistency, is of poor reliability and validity and is of limited use for establishing baselines, defining standards, making comparisons or tracking trends' (UNISDR 2011b, p. 46).

This statement relates to a report, published under the auspices of ISDR on 'Evidence for disaster risk management', which offers scientific processes for information and knowledge needs for policy makers and field practitioners (Murray et al. 2011). This report concluded that evidence is imperative for strengthening all aspects of disaster risk management. It went onto to state that 'the HFA Mid Term Review could encourage greater national and international investments in standardised collection and use of high-quality data, information and evidence to set up relevant baselines before events occur and ensure that tools used in disaster risk management can be evaluated against agreed benchmarks' (Murray et al. 2011, pp. 9–10). Finally it finished by stating that 'data, information and knowledge management are critical measures for saving lives and reducing suffering of people at risk of or affected by emergencies disasters' (Murray et al. 2011, p. 10).

10.5 Conclusions

Natural and man-made disasters can be humanitarian catastrophes, with significant morbidity and mortality. Undertaking health and social research to help facilitate disaster risk reduction and disaster risk management is vitally important to increase preparedness to respond to disasters, to enable the most effective action to be taken once disasters have occurred and to understand better the consequences of disasters.

In this chapter we have considered the setting of disaster research priorities. We have examined three of the possible approaches to the setting of disaster research priorities, and considered ethical issues pertaining to these approaches: the example of priority setting in the healthcare context; how disaster research priorities have been developed by organisations involved in disaster response; and a UN-endorsed strategic approach to disaster risk management stemming from the Hyogo Framework for Action.

None of these approaches is comprehensive but each provides, in different ways, helpful frameworks for considering the setting of disaster research priorities. Taken together, we hope that they will provide a platform for further thinking and action to develop ethical and effective ways of setting priorities in this difficult but vital area.

References

Anand, Sudhir., Fabienne Peter., and Amartya Sen. 2004. *Public health, ethics, and equity*. Oxford: Oxford University Press.

Daniels, Norman., and James E. Sabin. 1997. Limits to health care: Fair procedures, democratic deliberation and the legitimacy problem for insurers. *Philo Pub Affairs* 26(4):303–502.

Daniels, Norman. 2000. Accountability for reasonableness: Establishing a fair process for priority setting is easier than agreeing on principles. *BMJ* 321:1300–1301.

Daniels, Norman., and James E. Sabin. 2008. Accountability for reasonableness: an update. *BMJ* 337:1850.

Elliot, A.J, N. Singh., P. Loveridge., S. Harcourt., S. Smith., R. Pnaiser., K. Kavanagh., C. Robertson., C.N. Ramsay., J. McMenamin., A. Kibble., V. Murray., S. Ibbotson., M. Catchpole., B. McCloskey., and G.E. Smith. 2010. Syndromic surveillance to assess the potential public health impact of the Icelandic volcanic ash plume across the United Kingdom. *Eurosurveillance* 15(23). http://www.eurosurveillance.org/ViewArticle.aspx?ArticleId=19583. Accessed 6 November 2011.

Enhanced Learning and Research for Humanitarian Aid ELRHA. 2011a. About us. http://www.elrha.org/about. Accessed 29 September 2011.

Enhanced Learning and Research for Humanitarian Aid ELRHA. 2011b. Humanitarian Principles. http://www.elrha.org/?q=node/89. Accessed 29 September 2011.

Gibson, J., D. Martin, and P. Singer. 2002. Priority setting for new technologies in medicine: A transdisciplinary study. *BMC Health Services Research* 2:14 doi:10.1186/1472-6963-2-14.

Gruskin, S., and N. Daniels. 2008. Justice and human rights: Priority setting and fair, deliberative process. *Am J Pub Health* 98:1573–7.

Health Protection Agency (HPA). 2010. Strategic overview 2010–2015. Preparing, preventing, responding. http://www.hpa.org.uk/web/HPAwebFile/HPAweb_C/1274087971865. Accessed 30 September 2011.

Health Protection Agency (HPA). 2011a. Annual report and accounts 2010/11. http://www.hpa.org.uk/webc/HPAwebFile/HPAweb_C/1296689072996. Accessed 6 November 2011.

Health Protection Agency (HPA). 2011b. Extreme Events and Health Protection Section (EEHPS). http://www.hpa.org.uk/AboutTheHPA/WhoWeAre/CentreForRadiationChemicalAndEnvironmentalHazards/crceEEHPSdescription/. Accessed 30 September 2011.

Hughes, D. A., B. Tunnage., and S. T. Yeo. 2005. Drugs for exceptionally rare diseases: Do they deserve special status for funding? *QJM* 98:829–836.

Imperial College and King's College London (IC/KCL). 2011. MRC-HPA centre for environment & health. Centre mission statement. http://www.environment-health.ac.uk/Mission.aspx Accessed 30 September 2011.

Intergovernmental Panel on Climate Change (IPCC). 2009. Scoping meeting for an IPCC special report on extreme events and disasters: Managing the risks. https://www.ipcc-wg1.unibe.ch/srex/SREX-Oslo_Proceedings_Final.pdf. Accessed 6 November 2011.

Intergovernmental Panel on Climate Change (IPCC). 2012. Managing the risks of extreme events and disasters to advance climate change adaptation. Special report of the intergovernmental panel on climate change. http://ipcc-wg2.gov/SREX/. Accessed 1 June 2013.

International Council for Science (ICSU). 2003. ICSU Report of the CSPR assessment panel on environment and its relation to sustainable Development. http://www.icsu.org/publications/reports-and-reviews/priority-area-assessment-on-environment-and-its-relation-to-sustainable-development/ICSU_PAA_REPORT.pdf. Accessed 17 February 2011.

International Council for Science (ICSU). 2004. Foresight analysis. http://www.icsu.org/publications/reports-and-reviews/foresight-analysis/Foresight-Analysis.pdf. Accessed 17 February 2011.

International Council for Science (ICSU). 2006. ICSU report of the CSPR assessment panel on capacity building in science. http://www.icsu.org/publications/reports-and-reviews/paa-capacity-building/PAA-Cap-Building.pdf. Accessed 17 February 2011.

International Council for Science (ICSU). 2008. A science plan for integrated research on disaster risk: Addressing the challenge of natural and human-induced environmental hazards. http://www.icsu.org/publications/reports-and-reviews/IRDR-science-plan/irdr-science-plan.pdf. Accessed 26 November 2010.

Kovats,Sari R., Helen, Johnson., and Clare, Griffiths. 2006. Mortality in southern England during the 2003 heat wave by place of death. *Health Stat Quart* 29:6–8. http://ons.gov.uk/ons/search/index.html?newquery=mortality+in+southern+england+the+2003+heatwave. Accessed 6 November 2011.

Maiese, Michelle. 2003. Distributive justice. http://www.beyondintractability.org/bi-essay/distributive-justice. Accessed 6 November 2011.

McKie, John, and Jeff Richardson. 2003. The rule of rescue. *Soc Sci Med* 56:2407–2419.

Médecins, Sans Frontières (MSF). 2005. Ethics Review Board. Ethics framework for medical research. http://fieldresearch.msf.org/msf/handle/10144/12364. Accessed 6 November 2011.

Murray, Virginia., Ishani Kar-Purkayastha., Delphine Grynzpan., Jonathan Abrahams., and Altaf Musani. 2011. Evidence for disaster risk management—Information and knowledge needs for policy makers and field practitioners. United Nations international strategy for disaster reduction hyogo framework for action mid term review, Global Platform. http://www.unisdr.org/files/18197_205murray.evidencefordisasterriskma.pdf. Accessed 6 November 2011.

National Commission for the Protection of Human Subjects of Biomedical and Behavioral Research (NCPHSBBR). 1979. *The Belmont Report. Ethical principles and guidelines for the protection of human subjects of research*. Washington, DC: US Government Printing Office.

National Institute for Health and Clinical Excellence (NICE). 2008. Social value judgments: principles for the development of NICE guidance. www.nice.org.uk/aboutnice/howwework/socialvaluejudgements/socialvaluejudgements.jsp. Accessed 6 November 2011.

National Institute for Health and Clinical Excellence (NICE). 2010. Capecitabine for the treatment of advanced gastric cancer. http://www.nice.org.uk/nicemedia/live/13049/49875/49875.pdf. Accessed 6 November 2011.

National Institute for Health and Clinical Excellence (NICE). 2011. Pazopanib for the first-line treatment of advanced renal cell carcinoma. http://www.nice.org.uk/nicemedia/live/13346/53304/53304.pdf. Accessed 6 November 2011.

Pitt, Michael. 2008. The Pitt Review: Lessons learned from the 2007 floods. UK Cabinet Office. http://webarchive.nationalarchives.gov.uk/20100807034701/http:/archive.cabinetoffice.gov.uk/pittreview/thepittreview.html. Accessed 6 November 2011.

Rhodes, Rosamond., Margaret P. Battin., and Anita Silvers, eds. 2002. *Medicine and social justice: Essays on the distribution of health care*. Oxford: Oxford University Press.

Sheather, Julian., and Tejshri, Shah. 2011. Ethical dilemmas in medical humanitarian practice: Cases for reflection from Médecins Sans Frontières. *J Med Eth* 37:162–165.

UK HM Government. Health Protection Agency Act 2004. http://www.legislation.gov.uk/ukpga/2004/17/contents. Accessed 6 November 2011.

United Nations International Strategy on Disaster Reduction (UNISDR). 2007. Hyogo Framework for Action: Building the Resilience of Nations and Communities to Disasters 2005–2015. http://www.unisdr.org/files/1037_hyogoframeworkforactionenglish.pdf. Accessed 6 November 2011.

United Nations International Strategy on International Strategy for Disaster Reduction (UNISDR). Science and Technical Committee. 2009a. Reducing disaster risks through science: Issues and actions. Report from the second session of the Global Platform for Disaster Risk Reduction in Geneva, 16–19 June 2009. http://www.preventionweb.net/globalplatform/2009/background/documents/SD-03-ENG-Scientific-Technical-Committee.pdf. Accessed 17 February 2011.

United Nations International Strategy on Disaster Reduction (UNISDR). Science and Technical Committee. 2009b. Reducing disaster risks through science: Issues and Actions. http://www.unisdr.org/preventionweb/files/11543_STCReportlibrary.pdf. Accessed 17 February 2011.

United Nations International Strategy for Disaster Reduction (UNISDR). 2011a. Who we are. http://www.unisdr.org/eng/about_isdr/isdr-mission-objectives-eng.htm. Accessed 6 November 2011.

United Nations International Strategy on Disaster Reduction (UNISDR). 2011b. Hyogo Framework for Action 2005–2015. Building the resilience of nations and communities to disasters. Mid-term review 2010–2011. http://www.unisdr.org/files/18197_midterm.pdf. Accessed 6 November 2011.

Weber, Heike, and Caroline, Culshaw. 2009. Workshop on environmental exposure and health. Medical Research Council and Natural Environment Research Council. http://www.nerc.ac.uk/research/programmes/eehi/documents/eeh-workshop-report.pdf. Accessed 30 September 2011.

World Health Organisation, Health Protection Agency, United Nations International Strategy on Disaster Reduction (WHO/HPA/UNISDR). 2011. Disaster risk management for health advocacy sheets. http://www.hpa.org.uk/Topics/EmergencyResponse/ExtremeWeatherEventsAndNaturalDisasters/DisasterRiskManagementFactsheets/ and http://www.who.int/hac/events/disaster_reduction_2011/en. Accessed 6 November 2011.

Chapter 11
Studying Vulnerable Populations in the Context of Enhanced Vulnerability

Ruth Macklin

Brief portions of this article are excerpted from my previously published works: Macklin, Ruth. Double standards in medical research in developing countries. 2004. Cambridge, U.K.: Cambridge University Press; Macklin, Ruth. Ethics and clinical research. 2010. Barcelona, Spain: Fundació Víctor Grífols i Lucas; Macklin, Ruth and Ethan Cowan. 2009. Conducting research in disease outbreaks, PLoS Neglected Tropical Diseases 3:1–3.

11.1 Critiquing the Need for Research

Arguments critical of research conducted in disasters focus on one or more of the following points: 1) victims in the midst of a disaster are rendered too vulnerable by the situation to permit their inclusion in research; 2) natural disasters or disease outbreaks in developing countries or poor areas in industrialised countries render the inhabitants even more vulnerable, since what they need is aid, not research; 3) people who are recruited by health workers during a disaster may confuse research with treatment and fall prey to the therapeutic misconception; 4) people caught in a disaster are too emotionally unstable to provide valid informed consent to be a research subject; 5) even following a disaster, those caught in its wake may be traumatised by interviews or physical examinations that cause them to recall terrible circumstances; 6) conducting research in a disaster may impede efforts to mitigate harm and can intrude into rescue operations; and 7) when disaster strikes there is insufficient time to prepare a proper research protocol and have it reviewed by a research ethics committee, so potential subjects may lack adequate protection of their rights and welfare. Responses to these criticisms require a deeper inquiry into the concept of vulnerability, a look at what empirical evidence shows about the mental and emotional state of individuals caught up in disasters, and careful planning to avoid the problems noted in the above criticisms.

R. Macklin (✉)
Albert Einstein College of Medicine, Bronx, New York, USA
e-mail: ruth.macklin@einstein.yu.edu

D. P. O'Mathúna et al. (eds.), *Disaster Bioethics: Normative Issues When Nothing is Normal,* Public Health Ethics Analysis 2, DOI 10.1007/978-94-007-3864-5_11,

11.2 The Need for Research in Disasters

It would take an encyclopaedic volume to describe all the circumstances in various types of disasters where research is needed that can inform better actions in the future. The authors of an article discussing the need for research during or after a terrorist attack provide the following reasons: 'Research that focuses on the effects of terrorism can provide important information that may improve long-term survival, help prepare for subsequent incidents, assess the physical and emotional needs of a population, have an impact on mental health management of victims and other disaster-affected persons, and increase understanding of the human experience' (Fleischman and Wood 2002, p. 315). Three additional illustrations provide more specific details.

The first is a rather technical example regarding exposure to radiation in accidents. The second is a somewhat neglected area: sex and gender differences in vulnerability to disasters and their impact. The third is how best to manage compound fractures and crush injuries in disasters such as earthquakes, which cause many limb fractures.

The authors of a scientific article on accidental radiation exposure begin with the sobering observation that in today's world, there is an enhanced likelihood of accidental radiation exposure to occupational workers, patients and the public (Pandey et al. 2010). Citing the increasing use of nuclear technology in power production, medical and industrial applications, and the possibility of nuclear terrorism or war, the authors describe current knowledge and necessary additional research to improve the treatment and management of victims of radiation accidents. Among other areas where research during radiation accidents can contribute to existing scientific understanding, the article notes that 'there is a need to fill the gaps in knowledge of radiation action in different dose ranges and post-irradiation windows, which would help in improving therapeutic approaches' (Pandey et al. 2010, p. 613). What is striking about the information in the article—at least to a layperson in the field of radiation—are the myriad differences between types of exposure to large doses of radiation. To cite only one example: the radiation exposure from the Chernobyl nuclear accident differed markedly from what the population in Hiroshima and Nagasaki experienced from the atomic bombings. In the atomic bombings, people were exposed to external whole body radiation and minimal exposure from fallout of the radioisotopes. In contrast, in Chernobyl 'millions of people were exposed to a significant level of radioactivity from fallout and external radiation; however, whole body exposure was limited to those working close to the reactor or post-accidental rescue workers' (Pandey et al. 2010, p. 613). Because of these and other differences, the article notes that the expected health consequences to the victims of the Chernobyl accident would be different from those for the atomic bombs survivors. This article was published in August 2010, less than a year before the effects of the earthquake and tsunami devastated the Fukushima Daiichi nuclear plant in Japan. But one can imagine that the circumstances for workers and the public there would differ yet again from those in Chernobyl in 1986 and in Hiroshima and Nagasaki in 1945. After presenting a staggering amount of data on reactions of the human body to an array of radioactive substances, Pandey et al. issue a few caveats regarding research during a disaster. One is that casualties of radiation accidents may require the screening of large numbers of individuals—a practical limitation. Other limiting factors are high cost, sophisticated machines, need for trained personnel, and lack of established biomarkers specific to radiation. If we contemplate how clinical studies could practicably have been conducted in the wake of the March 2011 earthquake and tsunami in Japan, the likelihood of such highly sophisticated research appears slim indeed. However, if exposure of large numbers of people occurs near one or more tertiary care hospitals, it may be possible to conduct research while attending scrupulously to the needs of the exposed individuals.

A second illustration is provided by a World Health Organization (WHO) report that noted 'There is a general lack of research on sex and gender differences in vulnerability to and impact of disasters' (World Health Organization 2002). In all likelihood, not much has changed in the intervening decade. Mentioning the limited amount of existing evidence, WHO reported differences between women and men in the negative consequences following a disaster. It is not clear, the report states, whether these are a result of biological differences, socially determined differences, or some combination of the two. Citing an array of statistics and anecdotes, the WHO report paints a picture of greater vulnerability of women than men when disasters strike. The WHO report describes an earthquake in Maharashtra, India, where many more women died than men. Women were inside homes that collapsed, while men were in the open fields during harvest time and boys were away at schools distant from the site of the earthquake. Regarding another well-known phenomenon, the report says that 'Women and girls are more vulnerable to sexual abuse in disaster situations and may be coerced into sex for basic needs such as food, shelter and security. The sex industry often becomes part of the interaction between the refugee or displaced population and the local community' (World Health Organization 2002). Despite these and numerous other known circumstances differentiating the consequences of disasters for women and men, WHO points to the need for additional research at local, national, and international levels. At the local level, research is needed on how gender relations operate in households and communities in a disaster situation and during the relief and recovery phase. Another area that needs to be better researched in the wake of disasters is the special needs of disadvantaged women, such as women with disabilities and women in violent relationships. Even within disaster organisations, studies are needed to determine the effects of gendered organisational culture on staffing, funding, programming, and training. This WHO report is an eye-opening reminder that even in the 21st century, there remains substantial neglect of the type of research that addresses gender equity in situations such as disasters.

A third area where research is needed is how best to manage compound fractures and crush injuries in disasters such as earthquakes, which typically cause many such injuries. Compound fractures may be able to be managed by fixation. Open fractures are typically considered lethal unless they are treated because the open limb is exposed to infection (Rajpura et al. 2010). Under ideal circumstances, treatment is surgical fixation followed by a recovery period. For a large group of victims whose limbs are severely affected, amputation above the injury is most likely to save lives. It is clearly more efficient in a disaster setting than surgical fixation, and would undoubtedly cost less. However, if local hospitals have the personnel and facilities, it may be possible to do either procedure, presenting the opportunity to study survival, effectiveness, time to recovery, and cost-effectiveness. Arguably, it would be unethical to randomise patients into a surgical fixation group or an amputation group. This is because people have strong preferences about the value they place on continued life versus living with a disability. Some would clearly choose amputation with a better chance of survival, whereas others would prefer to take their chances with surgical fixation in order to save the limb. If they are able to consent, they might be given a choice of treatment, but could still be studied in comparison groups. This would have the usual consequence of potential bias in studies comparing two groups that are not randomised. However, if there were enough victims of injury who are truly indifferent regarding the two procedures and their different probable outcomes, and are willing to consent to be randomised, then the optimal research design could be used. In addition to the usual problems surrounding informed consent in a disaster, these victims may lack the capacity to consent. For those individuals, a decision still has to be made about which of the available treatments to undertake. Their preference would be unknown, so presumably the intervention more likely to save lives would be the one physicians should choose. Those patients could still be used as a comparison group for those who have capacity and make their own choice.

One of the most ethically problematic and emotional wrenching features of a medical response to a disaster is the need for triage. Victims whose condition is so serious that survival is highly unlikely are triaged out of a medical treatment group. Those who have both open fractures and a crush injury are likely to be triaged out; yet data may be gathered regarding their condition as part of the emergency response: time to death, and other information that may be useful in determining the appropriateness of triage for similar victims in the future. The prospect of gathering such information without obtaining consent appears to violate the most basic principle of research ethics. However, if observations and recording such data is considered part of a public health emergency preparedness and response, it would be perfectly acceptable. A variety of interventions may be necessary for victims of crush injuries, depending on what facilities are available. Hypotension, renal failure, metabolic abnormalities, and secondary complications are some of the medical consequences that can be managed in a hospital setting (Centers for Disease Control and Prevention 2011).

Given the large numbers of victims of an earthquake who could be studied in comparison groups where the best management is uncertain or disputed, thereby satisfying the requirement of clinical equipoise, research could yield valuable information for similar circumstances in the future. That a hospital setting can be available even when an earthquake strikes in a resource-poor country is demonstrated by the field hospital set up by the Israel Defense Forces Medical Corps in Haiti within 89 hours of the earthquake in January 2010 (Kreiss et al. 2010). It remains true, however, that if one set of best practices is implemented and studied, it could be categorised as an emergency response, part of typical public health practice; but if patients are randomised into comparison groups, it immediately qualifies as research, with all the procedural safeguards and protections that entails–especially the requirement of informed consent. If ever there were a situation in which research appears to be ethically permissible without obtaining informed consent, it is in a disaster where clinical equipoise exists and the victims are incapable of giving their informed consent to be studied.

11.3 Vulnerability in Disaster Settings

The single best justification for conducting research in the midst or in the wake of a disaster is captured by the following statement: 'To ensure effective and equitable responses to future disasters, we need to study what works and what doesn't work in present disasters' (Public Health Ethics in Disasters 2011). However, without devoting attention to the ethical concerns posed by the conduct of research in disasters, this justification is too simplistic. The first step is to address the threshold question: 1) Are victims of a disaster rendered too vulnerable by the situation to permit their inclusion in research (O'Mathúna 2010)? One reason this question is hard to answer is that there is no clear, universally accepted criterion for applying the concept of vulnerability. Let's take a brief look at what several international ethical guidance documents say about vulnerable subjects of research.

The *Declaration of Helsinki* is probably the best known document regarding ethics in research with human beings. However, its description of vulnerable subjects is both narrow and brief: 'Some research populations are particularly vulnerable and need special protection. These include those who cannot give or refuse consent for themselves and those who may be vulnerable to coercion or undue influence' (World Medical Association 2008 Para. 9). These characteristics of vulnerability appear more applicable to clinical research, where patients are the research subjects, than to the majority of people caught in a disaster. In addition, the description of vulnerability is too general to provide concrete guidance. What 'special protections' are appropriate or necessary? What specific features determine the ability of people to give or refuse consent? What sort of coercion might be present?

Although little empirical evidence exists regarding the extent to which people in disaster situations are vulnerable to coercion, one article gives this limited information: '[I]n a study of trauma survivors who were asked to participate in a clinical study, 19% of subjects endorsed the statement "I felt like I couldn't say no to participating" ' (Rosenstein 2004, p. 376). But the author of the article goes on to note that there was no comparison group in this study, and it is not possible to know if the subjects' unwillingness to refuse participation was specifically related to their having been traumatised. Still, when research is carried out in a disaster side by side with delivery of humanitarian aid, individuals may feel pressured to participate if they hold the (false) belief that assistance is contingent on their agreement to participate in research (O'Mathúna 2010).

The Council for International Organizations of Medical Sciences (CIOMS) *International Ethical Guidelines for Biomedical Research* include a guideline entitled

'Research involving vulnerable persons', which states 'Special justification is required for inviting vulnerable individuals to serve as research subjects and, if they are selected, the means of protecting their rights and welfare must be strictly applied' (CIOMS 2002, p. 64). The individuals or groups mentioned in the guideline are identified as follows: 'Vulnerable persons are those who are relatively (or absolutely) incapable of protecting their own interests. More formally, they may have insufficient power, intelligence, education, resources, strength, or other needed attributes to protect their own interests' (p. 64). The chief characteristic of vulnerability this guideline identifies is a limited capacity or freedom to consent or to decline to participate in research. The criterion of 'limited freedom to consent' does not seem particularly relevant to individuals in a disaster, but some individuals may have limited capacity because of trauma, stress, or injury. The commentary following the CIOMS guideline lists numerous specific groups that may be considered vulnerable in the context of research. These include subordinate members of hierarchical groups, such as the military or students; elderly persons with dementia and residents of nursing homes; people receiving welfare benefits or social assistance, other poor people, and the unemployed; patients in emergency rooms; some ethnic and racial minority groups; homeless persons, nomads, refugees or displaced persons; prisoners; patients with incurable disease; individuals who are politically powerless; and members of communities unfamiliar with modern medical concepts. The CIOMS guideline makes no mention of victims of disasters. Members of some of the above-mentioned groups may be caught in a disaster, such as elderly residents of nursing homes when Hurricane Katrina struck in New Orleans in 2005 (Khanna et al. 2005), and some people in rural areas of Japan affected by the earthquake and tsunami in March 2011. However, many people who do not fit into any of the above categories also lose their lives or are seriously injured in disasters.

Still another list of vulnerable populations appears in an ethical guidance document specific to HIV biomedical prevention research: 'Examples of populations that may have an increased vulnerability include women, children and adolescents, men who have sex with men, injecting drug users, sex workers, transgender persons, indigenous populations, the poor, the homeless, and communities from resource-poor settings in high-income and low- and middle-income countries' (UNAIDS/WHO 2007, p. 31). In this document, like the others, there is no mention of people who are caught in a disaster situation.

These various accounts of vulnerable research subjects have prompted some scepticism and a bit of a backlash regarding overuse of the concept of vulnerability. The scepticism is whether all of these various groups really should be considered vulnerable. If so, for what reason and what are the implications for involving them in research? The backlash questions whether the concept of vulnerability actually makes sense when there are so many candidates, thus prompting the question, 'Who is not vulnerable?' According to one article, 'So many groups are now considered to be vulnerable in the context of research, particularly international research, that the concept has lost force' (Levine et al. 2004, p. 44). The authors add: '... so many categories of people are now considered vulnerable that virtually all potential human subjects are included' (Levine et al. 2004, p. 46).

Among the prominent ethical concerns about conducting research during or after disasters are those related to stress, trauma, and the ability of victims to provide informed consent (Rosenstein 2004; O'Mathúna 2010). One author concludes: 'There are no compelling data to suggest that experiencing a severe trauma, in and of itself, renders all or even most exposed individuals incapable of making autonomous decisions' (Rosenstein 2004, p. 373). If there is difficulty ascertaining individuals' capacity to provide informed consent to participate in disaster research, there is little reason to believe the problem is worse than what exists in the clinical setting. For example, the presumption in research involving psychiatric patients is that they are capable of consenting to research; evidence to the contrary must be presented if such patients are to be excluded (Appelbaum and Roth 1982). Some studies involving psychiatric patients or those who appear demented require an evaluation of individuals' capacity before they may be enrolled in research. The same procedure could be adopted in cases where doubt exists about the capacity of potential subjects in disaster research. From a practical point of view, however, this procedure would be difficult to implement when researchers seek to interview people in the chaos and confusion that typically accompany a disaster.

A different but related concern is whether individuals involved in extremely traumatic situations can anticipate the distress or discomfort they may experience as participants in disaster research (Collogan et al. 2004). Here again, the analogy with clinical and behavioural research is apt. Patients who have never undergone an invasive medical procedure as part of their medical care may nevertheless be invited to participate in a research study related to their medical condition. The procedure may cause a degree of pain or discomfort they could not foresee merely by reading or hearing the description provided in the informed consent process or document. Participants in sensitive social science research on sexuality and reproductive health or intimate partner violence are typically informed that some questions are sensitive and may make them feel uncomfortable. Yet the experience of being asked and answering such questions may provoke feelings the potential subject did not anticipate. Collogan and colleagues make a sharp distinction between trauma caused by the disaster itself, and the feelings participants in research may have when those events are recalled: 'Research participation may upset subjects but it does not traumatize them as a disastrous event would. Trauma-inducing events involve unpredictable and uncontrollable experiences, while disaster-focused research should be both predictable and highly controlled' (Collogan et al. 2004, p. 367).

The bioethics literature includes two articles that make useful distinctions when considering research involving disaster victims. The first distinction is that between 'intrinsic' and 'extrinsic' vulnerability. Intrinsic vulnerability refers to factors such as increased age, extreme youth, decreased cognitive ability, or psychosis. Extrinsic vulnerability refers to situations such as hospitalisation, imprisonment, or financial capacity (Dean and McClement 2002). According to this distinction, the large majority, if not all of the people caught in the wake of a disaster share the characteristic of 'extrinsic vulnerability.' Among that group, the elderly, infants and young children, people with physical, mental, or emotional disabilities are also 'intrinsically vulnerable.' This may be useful in determining which individuals or groups it is more or less ethically acceptable to involve in research during or after a disaster. The appropriateness also depends on the type of research, an additional factor noted below.

A second useful distinction in considering research with vulnerable populations introduces the idea of 'layers of vulnerability' (Luna 2009). According to Luna:

> This concept of vulnerability is a relational one. That is, it concerns the relation between the person or a group of persons and the circumstances or the context. It is closely related to the situation under analysis. It is not a category or a label we can just put on ... If this is so, vulnerability should not be understood as a permanent and categorical condition, a label that is attached to someone given certain conditions (such as lack of power or incapability) that persists throughout its existence ... The proposal based on layers has a related advantage. It can help in making a refined analysis of research situations. (Luna 2009, p. 129)

How would the 'layers' approach apply to the vulnerability of people caught in a disaster? The answer depends on the condition of the individuals and the nature of the research. The condition of individuals is likely to vary with the type and severity of the disaster and their exposure to harmful effects. People who are physically injured in an earthquake, for example, may be traumatised or in pain. First responders, such as fire-fighters, may be overcome by smoke or, as in the case of the terrorist attack in New York on September 11, 2001, exposed to huge quantities of dust from the collapsing buildings. People who receive very large doses of radiation may suffer immediate ill effects, as in the Chernobyl and Fukushima Daiichi nuclear plant disasters. Individuals who fall ill in an infectious disease outbreak, such as the SARS and H1N1 influenza epidemics may be too sick to answer questions or consent to provide blood samples. The characteristic of 'extrinsic vulnerability' applies to all these groups. An additional 'layer' of vulnerability would result from 'intrinsic' factors such as infirmity, disability, poor nutritional status, or an underlying disease.

The nature of the research also varies considerably. Much research conducted during or soon after a disaster is social science research: surveys, questionnaires, or in-depth interviews. This type of investigation is usually categorised as 'minimal risk' research, which is defined as involving risks of a scale ordinarily encountered in daily life or during the performance of routine physical or psychological examinations or tests' (US Department of Health and Human Services 2009 46.102(h)(i)). The harms likely to befall individuals who are asked to participate are emotional stress and invasions of their privacy by asking intrusive questions. Another type of research likely to occur in disasters such as disease outbreaks and radiation exposure involves drawing blood, also normally considered minimal risk research. Where the risks to research participants are minimal, concerns about vulnerability are a function of the ability of the subjects to consent, and not to their exposure to risks of a potentially harmful medication. On the other hand, investigations of new drugs or experimental use of existing medications to study antidotes in people exposed to attacks of anthrax or other biological agents would constitute more than minimal risk because of known side effects or unknown harmful effects. This last situation best demonstrates the 'layers' approach to vulnerability: disaster victims may be exposed to toxic or even lethal substances, they may be sick or debilitated from that exposure, and the research intervention itself carries some risks of harm and unanticipated adverse events.

Past studies have revealed several characteristics of participants and types of studies in which disaster research has increased the subjects' potential for experiencing harms. 'These characteristics include pre-existing distress or mental illness, age (both young and old), history of multiple trauma exposures, social vulnerability, and physical injury. Furthermore, evidence suggests that repetitive research involving the same participants carries a potential for risk' (Collogan et al. 2004, p. 367). Many investigators would like to study people who have direct exposure to a particular disaster. Such individuals may be overburdened with requests to be interviewed, thereby confronting painful memories and feelings repeatedly. An enhanced potential for experiencing harms can translate into greater vulnerability, again illustrating the value of the 'layers' approach. One or more of the above characteristics of participants or types of studies can be considered an additional 'layer.' With this concept, the notion of vulnerability loses much of its vagueness and becomes more meaningful for determining what steps might be needed to protect the rights and welfare of participants in disaster research.

I contend that even where a credible case can be made that potential subjects of research are vulnerable— by using the 'layers' approach—this should not be a barrier to conducting the research. The situation is no different, in principle, from much biomedical or social science research in more usual circumstances. Medical research is conducted on severely ill patients, including those with fatal illnesses such as end-stage cancer, degenerative neuromuscular conditions, and Alzheimer's disease. When cancer patients become subjects in research they are exposed to toxic chemotherapy, drugs with significant side effects, and radiation treatment. Social science research is carried out on victims of intimate partner violence, women who have been raped, and soldiers returning from embattled war zones with post-traumatic stress disorder (PTSD). Unless all these types of research are unethical and should not be conducted because participants have layers of vulnerability, doing research in situations of disaster should not be considered unique based on the vulnerability of the subject population. As already noted, 'we need to study what works and what doesn't work' in order to prepare properly for future disasters. The authors of one article add: 'Although the risks and benefits of participation in disaster-focused research are not fully understood, most would agree that there is a significant need for additional research in the aftermath of disaster' (Collogan et al. 2004, p. 364).

The ethical guidelines for research mentioned earlier raise the question whether inhabitants of resource-poor countries are particularly vulnerable, due to poverty, their lack of accessibility to routine health care, or the poor infrastructure in the country. Do natural disasters or disease outbreaks in developing countries or poor areas in industrialised countries render the inhabitants even more vulnerable, since what they need is aid, not research (O'Mathúna 2010)? It is unquestionably true that the 2010 earthquake in Haiti, Hurricane Katrina in 2005 in New Orleans, and the 2008 earthquake in China did more damage and resulted in more loss of lives than similar events in wealthier countries or communities and in places with a far better infrastructure. Individuals in resource-poor places lack money and often basic means of subsistence, and poor countries and communities take much longer to recover and begin providing necessary services to the inhabitants. Although barriers to resuming electricity, food and water supplies, and medical care were also formidable in the wake of the earthquake and tsunami in Japan, they are that much worse in resource-poor countries and communities. It is unquestionably true everywhere that the inhabitants and governments in places where earthquakes, hurricanes, monsoons, and tsunamis occur require huge amounts of governmental and humanitarian assistance from the outside. But this is not an either-or situation. The need for financial, medical, and other forms of aid should not be in competition with the conduct of research. The sources of research funding may be different, and the doctors, nurses, epidemiologists, and social scientists who carry out research are often not the same people as the providers of direct care.

11.4 Distinguishing Disaster Research from Public Health Practice

Not all research conducted during and after disasters involves human participants. Water and soil are often tested for contaminants and radioactive substances. Investigations of sources of infectious disease outbreaks take place in the environment or in buildings. Research goes on in laboratories far from the human beings affected. One circumstance that does involve human beings is problematic, however. That is, how to distinguish public health practice in response to disasters from research in the identical situation. Both activities require gathering data from people caught in the disaster. Both activities might involve drawing blood for detection of infection or radioactive material; and both activities could involve administering an antidote or medication and studying its effectiveness. A response to disasters considered to be public health practice is typically done under governmental authority, but can be conducted by humanitarian organisations such as Médecins Sans Frontières (MSF) and the International Red Cross. The purpose of the response is to document the existence and magnitude of a public health problem in a community or region and implement appropriate measures to deal with the problem.

The distinction between public health practice and public health research is not at all clear. It remains a "grey area" because of a conceptual problem in attempting to define 'research', and because of different criteria used by different groups to determine when a public health intervention is practice and when it is research (Calain 2009; Fairchild 2003). It is important, however, for practical and ethical reasons, to make the distinction. If an activity is research, an internationally accepted requirement is that it be submitted for prior review by a duly constituted, independent research ethics committee. In addition, a strong presumption exists that voluntary, informed consent be obtained from individuals who are invited to participate in research. In contrast, when a ministry of health or other branch of government at any level responds to a disaster, there is no need for prior review by a committee and no formal consent process when individuals are surveyed or interviewed. If blood drawing or medical treatment is involved, of course individuals must agree to cooperate, but there are no forms to read or sign and typically no detailed procedure to disclose risks, benefits, and alternatives. The uncertainty surrounding the distinction between public health practice and research can confuse researchers as well as people involved in a disaster who are approached by public health practitioners, physicians, social workers, social scientists, or those providing humanitarian assistance.

A widely accepted definition of 'research' is the following: '*Research* means a systematic investigation, including research development, testing and evaluation, designed to develop or contribute to generalisable knowledge' (US Department of Health and Human Services 2009). A key element in this definition is 'designed to contribute to knowledge that is generalisable.' The Centers for Disease Control and Prevention (CDC) in the United States uses a variation on this criterion for determining when an activity is research, referring to 'the primary intent' of the activity: 'If the primary intent is to prevent or control disease or injury or to improve a public health program, and no research is intended at the present time, the project is non-research' (Centers for Disease Control and Prevention 1999). One problem that arises for the ability to distinguish between public health response to emergencies and public health research is that what is learned in the course of the investigation may lead to generalisable knowledge, even if that was not the initial intent of the activity. A second problem is that the intent of an investigation is rarely specified in advance. As one article notes: '[T]o be credible, intents need to be specified in advance of potentially harmful activities, especially when very similar or identical activities are underpinned by different intents. This would imply the existence of independent bodies or agencies capable to record expressed intents ahead of the implementation of activities, a rather unrealistic proposal when applied to fast evolving emergency settings' (Calain 2009, p. 10).

Still another ethical problem arises when an emergency response contains elements of research in addition to the primary intent—to deal with the disaster situation. It may be an urgent response to the emergency with the usual public health purpose, and at the same time be an opportunity to conduct research that could lead to knowledge applicable to future similar situations. An example could be a questionnaire accompanied by drawing blood from people who become sick and those who remain well during a disease outbreak. At the same time that public health authorities take steps to slow the spread of the disease and protect uninfected people from becoming infected, they may seek to determine whether any biological, genetic, or life style factors caused some people to get sick while others did not. The effort to make such a determination qualifies as an intention to contribute to generalisable knowledge, and therefore as research. This situation is common when biological samples are stored for dual use during a disease outbreak, resulting in a mix of research and non-research (Calain 2009). According to regulations governing research in the United States, if these samples are anonymised at the time they are collected, the need for ethics committee review can be waived. However, this could not readily be done in the case of outbreaks such as Marburg and Ebola, as there is a need to match separate databases accurately, along with an obligation to communicate results to concerned individuals (Calain 2009).

In most cases in which there is an intent to conduct research, it requires preparation of a detailed research protocol. This would have to be submitted to the relevant research ethics committee for review and clearance, and the committee might request revision and resubmission of the protocol. This would delay the initiation of the response to the emergency, possibly resulting in greater harm to the population. In addition, conducting the activity as research would likely require obtaining informed consent from individuals for an activity as simple as a survey or short interview. This additional activity could take time and resources away from dealing directly with the emergency situation. If blood samples are sought from individuals, for example, to determine levels of radioactive substances, it is interesting to consider whether greater pressure could be exerted on them to allow their blood to be taken when the intervention is considered an emergency response than when it is clearly a research manoeuvre. In the latter case, the ethical requirement of the right of individuals to refuse to participate and not to be pressured or subjected to 'undue influence' should govern.

Regardless of whether a clear distinction can be made between gathering information for emergency response and gathering data for research, research ethics committees could establish a policy for disease outbreak investigations (Macklin and Cowan 2009). One possible element of the policy might be that investigators need not submit a full, detailed protocol to the committee at the outset of the study. The question of which research ethics committee(s) should be involved in approving such studies is a separate but related complication. The institution or organisation the researchers are from will almost always require ethical review, and international guidance documents typically require clearance by a local or national committee (CIOMS 2002). One or another committee could hold up the process, further delaying implementation of the research. A short statement of purpose and procedures of the investigation can be prepared and submitted for expedited review by a committee chair or other designated member. The CIOMS *International Ethical Guidelines for Epidemiological Studies* addresses this situation with the following observation: 'The emerging best practice for research conducted during emergency—such as population studies of outbreaks of disease or of disasters (and relief efforts)—is to establish the basic research design for various categories of research prior to the emergency. Among other benefits, this permits prior ethical review of at least the major features of the research design' (CIOMS 2009, p. 31). Even if an emergency response includes elements that unquestionably appear to be research, a duly constituted ethics oversight body could decide to waive the requirement for signed consent forms in favour of oral consent or even no consent from participants for interviews or surveys. This waiver could only be granted when the study is anonymous, that is, when individual participants cannot be identified and, as already noted, their consent must be obtained for collection of blood samples or other biological specimens.

Preparing in advance for conducting research during disease outbreaks or epidemics is not only possible, but appears to be easier than preparing in advance for research in other types of disaster. The enormous scale of destruction in earthquakes, tsunamis, and hurricanes may preclude a systematic study of the population involved. The unforeseen occurrence and suddenness of these natural events, as well as industrial disasters like the nuclear accident at Chernobyl and leakage of toxic chemicals at the Union Carbide pesticide plant in Bhopal, India, make it impossible to design a protocol for pre-approval by a research ethics committee. Nevertheless, a general outline or template can be prepared in advance for the predictable circumstances likely to arise in many disasters, such as the incidence of anxiety, the health consequences for displaced persons, and prevalence of PTSD. In all likelihood, the information gathered by local, regional, national, and international investigatory bodies will serve a dual purpose. Investigations in disasters serve the usual public health purpose of seeking to contain the disaster and mitigate its effects. And that information can be systematically recorded and analysed, and stored in a database, to be useful in similar circumstances in the future. Moreover, an investigation of some aspect of a disaster that begins as a public health response can transform into research as the inquiry develops. The CDC address this eventuality in its guidance on research and non-research: 'If the primary intent changes to generating generalizable knowledge, then the project becomes research' (Centers for Disease Control and Prevention 1999). This statement is an acknowledgment that the line between public health practice and public health research is fuzzy and can change as a response to a disaster evolves.

11.5 Conclusions

Whether research is contemplated at the outset of an emergency response to a disaster or is introduced at a later time, addressing questions related to the vulnerability of potential subjects remains an ethical requirement. One article observes that controversy exists over whether labelling a population as vulnerable may be stigmatising (Fleischman and Wood 2002). The authors correctly note that being vulnerable does not, in and of itself, raise the level of risk in a research study. However, vulnerable subjects deserve additional protections, even in research that would be categorised as 'minimal risk,' such as questionnaires or interviews. Ethical guidelines for research typically state the need for additional safeguards in the case of vulnerable subjects, but rarely specify what such protections should be. Different disasters may call for different safeguards for victims, depending on the proximity in time to the disaster in which the research takes place, the severity of injury or trauma, and other factors. When obtaining informed consent from victims in the aftermath of a disaster such as a terrorist attack, researchers should tell the subjects that the questions may be upsetting (Fleischman and Wood 2002). Similarly, researchers should plan in advance for serious emotional responses and have explicit mechanisms in place for referral to mental health professionals (Fleischman and Wood 2002). While this mechanism would almost certainly not be available for research carried out in places where there is widespread, severe damage and mental health professionals are busy attending to victims, it is feasible when survivors or relatives of people killed in the disaster are interviewed in the aftermath. In situations where there is time for a research ethics committee to review a proposal for a study, the committee could add procedural safeguards such as involvement of family members in the informed consent process and independent consent or research monitors (Fleischman and Wood 2002).

The types of safeguards needed for vulnerable subjects in research conducted during or after a disaster will depend on contextual factors that cannot be specified in advance. The "layers" approach to vulnerability can provide some guidance into additional protections for the rights and welfare of subjects that may be ethically necessary. One cardinal ethical principle that should always be adhered to is that research should never interfere with or delay medical care or other aid being provided to treat or prevent further harm to disaster victims.

References

Appelbaum, Paul S, and Loren H. Roth. 1982. Competency to consent to research: a psychiatric overview. *Archives of General Psychiatry* 39: 951–58.

Calain, Philippe. 2009. Research ethics and international epidemic response: the case of Ebola and Marburg hemorrhagic fevers. *Public Health Ethics* 2 (1): 7–29.

Centers for Disease Control and Prevention. 1999. Guidelines for defining public health research and public health non-research.1999. http://www.cdc.gov/od/science/integrity/docs/defining-public-health-research-non-research-1999.pdf. Accessed 3 May 2013.

Centers for Disease Control and Prevention. 2011. After an earthquake: management of crush injuries and crush syndrome. http://wwwnc.cdc.gov/travel/content/news-announcements/relief-workers-haiti.aspx. Accessed 9 May 2011.

CIOMS (Council for International Organizations of Medical Sciences). 2002. International ethical guidelines for biomedical research involving human subjects. http://cioms.ch/images/stories/CIOMS/guidelines/guidelines_nov_2002_blurb.htm. Accessed 4 May 2013.

CIOMS (Council for International Organizations of Medical Sciences). 2009. *International ethical guidelines on epidemiological studies. 2009*. Geneva, Switzerland: CIOMS.

Dean, Ruth A., and Susan E. McClement. 2002. Palliative care research: Methodological and ethical challenges. International *Journal of Palliative Nursing* 8 (8): 376–380.

Fairchild, Amy. 2003. Dealing with Humpty Dumpty: Research, practice, and the ethics of public health. *Journal of Law, Medicine, and Ethics* 31 (4): 615–623.

Fleischman, Alan R., and Emily B. Wood. 2002. Ethical issues in research involving victims of terror. *Journal of Urban Health* 79 (3): 315–321.

Fleischman, Alan R. 2004. Ethical issues pertaining to research in the aftermath of disaster. *Journal of Traumatic Stress* 17 (5): 363–372.

Khanna, Roma, Lise Olsen, and Anita Hassan. 2005. Storm evacuations: Elderly were left with weak safety net. Houston Chronicle, December 10.

Kreiss, Yitshak., Ofer Merin, Kobi Peleg, Gad Levy, Shlomo Vinker, Ram Sagi, Avi Abargel, Carmi Bartal, Guy Lin, Ariel Bar, Elhanan Bar-On, Mitchell J. Schwaber, and Nachman Ash. 2010. Early disaster response in Haiti: the Israeli field hospital experience. *Annals of Internal Medicine* 153 (1): 45–48.

Levine, Carole, Ruth Faden, Christine Grady, Dale Hammerschmidt, Lisa Eckenwiler, and Jeremy Sugarman. 2004. The limitations of "vulnerability" as a protection for human research participants. *The American Journal of Bioethics* 4 (3): 44–49.

Luna, Florencia. 2009. Elucidating the concept of vulnerability: layers not labels. *International Journal of Feminist Approaches to Bioethics* 2 (1): 121–139.

Macklin, Ruth, and Ethan Cowan. 2009. Conducting research in disease outbreaks. *PLoS Neglected Tropical Diseases* 3 (4): e335.

O'Mathúna, Dónal P. 2010. Conducting research in the aftermath of disasters: ethical considerations. *Journal of Evidence Based Medicine* 3 (2):65–75.

Pandey, Badri N., Amit Kumar, Prabha Tiwari, and Kaushala P. Mishra. 2010. Radiobiological basis in management of accidental radiation exposure. *International Journal of Radiation Biology* 86 (8): 613–35.

Public Health Ethics in Disasters. 2011. UNC Gillings school of global public health. Website accessed 9 May 2013 (no longer available).

Rajpura, Asim., Ihab Boutros, Tahir Khan, and Sohail A. Khan. 2010. Pakistan earthquake: experiences of a multidisciplinary surgical team. *Prehospital and Disaster Medicine* 25: 361–367.

Rosenstein, Donald L. 2004. Decision-making capacity and disaster research. *Journal of Traumatic Stress* 17 (5): 373–381.

UNAIDS/WHO. 2007. Ethical considerations in biomedical HIV prevention trials. http://www.unaids.org/en/media/unaids/contentassets/documents/unaidspublication/2012/jc1399_ethical_considerations_en.pdf. Accessed 4 May 2013.

US Department of Health and Human Services. 2009. Code of federal regulations: Protection of human subject. http://www.hhs.gov/ohrp/humansubjects/guidance/45cfr46.html. Accessed 4 May 2013.

World Health Organization. Gender and Health in Disasters. 2002. http://www.who.int/gender/other_health/en/genderdisasters.pdf. Accessed 3 May 2013.

World Medical Association. 2008. Declaration of Helsinki. http://www.wma.net/en/30publications/10policies/b3/. Accessed 4 May 2013.

Chapter 12
Research Ethics Governance in Disaster Situations

Doris Schopper

Given the deficit in international guidance about ethical oversight for emergency research and the fact that national regulations are frequently not adequate to govern ethical appraisal of research carried out in disaster-affected populations, an internationally recognised body should rapidly develop such guidance in collaboration with relevant organisations.

12.1 Introduction

A review of research on filovirus haemorrhagic fever outbreaks (Ebola/Marburg) published between 1999 and 2007, has shown that among 34 research interventions, individual consent was sought in fifteen cases and ethical review (international and local) was mentioned only in three cases (Calain et al. 2009). The paper also highlighted the deficit in international guidance about ethical issues when conducting research in epidemic emergencies. This chapter discusses the importance of such guidance and good ethics governance for research in disaster situations. There are several reasons why research ethics governance in disaster situations should receive special attention:

- Communities and people may be more vulnerable than under "normal" circumstances
- Research needs to be initiated quickly to be meaningful, in particular for the study community
- Normal oversight mechanisms may be unavailable in the country or region struck by the disaster
- Local research infrastructure may be seriously depleted or unavailable
- Research may involve (several) institutions or organisations from different parts of the world

D. Schopper (✉)
Center for Education and Research in Humanitarian Action,
University of Geneva, Geneva, Switzerland
e-mail: doris.schopper@unige.ch

D. P. O'Mathúna et al. (eds.), *Disaster Bioethics: Normative Issues When Nothing is Normal,* Public Health Ethics Analysis 2, DOI 10.1007/978-94-007-3864-5_12,

- The duty to provide emergency care may conflict with research priorities.

Some or all of these reasons may apply in various ways to research carried out during or after natural catastrophes such as Hurricane Katrina, the 2004 tsunami in South-East Asia, the 2010 earthquake in Haiti; man-made catastrophes such as Chernobyl, Fukushima, or Seveso; acute epidemics such as avian influenza, cholera, or Ebola/Marburg; and wars such as in Iraq, Afghanistan, or Somalia. Ethical scrutiny of research in emergency or post-emergency situations is paramount and has to abide by the same ethical principles as any research involving human subjects (Zwi et al. 2006). However, due to time constraints, ethics review procedures need to be particularly timely and flexible, and at the same time sufficiently stringent due to the potentially greater vulnerability of study communities (O'Mathúna 2010; Leaning 2001). Concern has also been voiced that research ethics boards may have limited experience regarding the protection of human subjects during a disaster (Fleischman and Wood 2002). This chapter will examine how these challenges can be addressed, using examples of review mechanisms which have been proposed and tried in various circumstances.

12.2 The Type of Research Influences the Review Procedure

The first question is what defines research involving human subjects in an emergency setting and would, therefore, require ethics review. Disaster research spans the spectrum from assessment of the initial situation (survey), evaluation of programmatic impact, testing new methods (laboratory devices, therapies, drugs), to clinical trials comparing different interventions, strategies or treatments (Ford et al. 2009). Research can be defined by its intention—to test a hypothesis, to generate new knowledge, to test a new intervention or one lacking evidence, or just to assess the need for intervention. Although everybody would agree that a randomised trial comparing the effectiveness of different drugs or an effectiveness evaluation of a novel surgical procedure is clearly research, there is much less agreement on, for example, nutrition or mortality surveys and assessments needed to monitor the implementation of a programme. How will it then be decided that ethics review is required and how stringent it has to be? The primordial question is whether there is potential harm to research participants and how considerable this potential harm can be. Based on a crude estimation of potential harm, a hierarchy of research going from minimal to great potential harm can be devised as shown in Fig. 12.1. The ethics review procedure and its stringency should then be commensurate with the type of research. How this can be envisaged and implemented in practice will be examined in more detail in sect. 12.3 and 12.4.

Expedited review is often mentioned as one mechanism to speed up the ethics review process in emergency research with various opinions on what this entails. For the purpose of this chapter, the following definition will be used: Expedited reviews are usually performed on a first come, first-served basis. Only one or two reviewers ensure that the protocol conforms to ethical standards and exercise oversight on

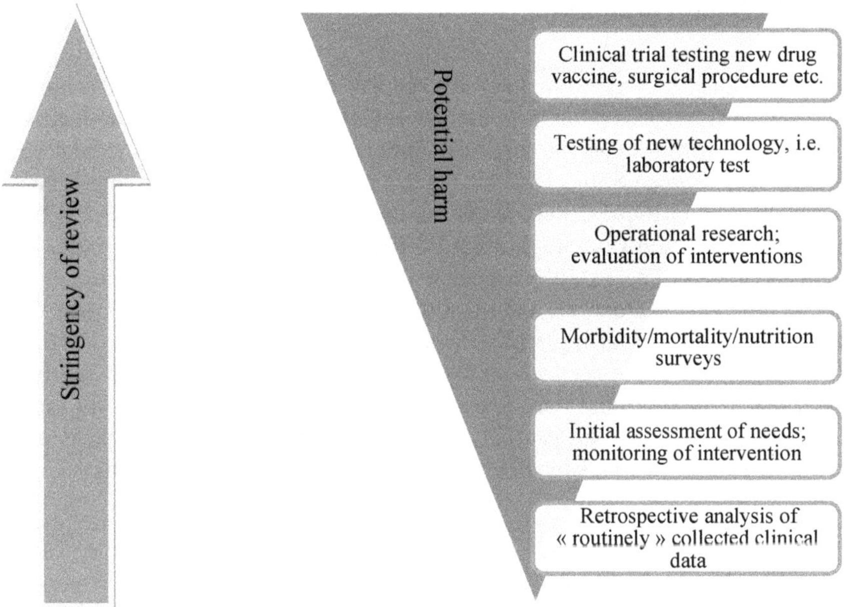

Fig. 12.1 Stringency of review procedure related to the type of research

behalf of the entire ethics review board. If a reviewer determines that a protocol does not meet specified conditions or has other concerns, he or she may remand the application to the full board. Only a full board can disapprove a study (Oakes 2002).

12.3 How Should Research Ethics Review be Adapted in Disaster Situations?

There are no agreed-upon international regulations governing ethics review for research carried out in the special circumstances of emergency interventions or disaster response. International, European and US regulations governing the ethics of medical research in emergency settings mainly focus on the issue of consent when they address such contexts specifically (Halila 2007; Calain et al. 2009). Given the dearth of guidance for ethics review of disaster research, several approaches have recently been proposed either embedded in broader ethics guidelines for research or examining explicitly the specific requirements for disaster research. Each will be described briefly to identify common threads or diverging propositions.

12.3.1 CIOMS Guidelines

The guidelines of the Council for International Organizations of Medical Sciences (CIOMS) are well respected and provide much valued guidance on research ethics including ethics review. The International Ethical Guidelines for Biomedical Research Involving Human Subjects (2002) make no explicit reference to emergency or disaster research (CIOMS 2002). However, the more recent edition of the CIOMS guidelines for epidemiological studies (CIOMS 2009) briefly addresses the issue. The commentary on guideline 2 ("Ethical review committees") includes a paragraph on research in emergency situations and mainly recommends establishing the research protocol beforehand, permitting prior ethical review of the main features of the research. It also points to the need for an expedient review process if no pre-approval has taken place. In addition, a commentary on guideline 6 ("Obtaining informed consent") suggests what to do if a person with an acute condition is incapable of giving informed consent. This may be relevant in certain disaster situations.

12.3.2 Tri-Council Policy Statement

The *Tri-Council Policy Statement: Ethical Conduct for Research Involving Humans* (TCPS) was jointly developed in 1998 by Canada's three federal research agencies. A revised edition, called TCPS 2, was published in 2010 after a large consultation process (Canadian Institutes of Health Research, Natural Sciences and Engineering Research Council of Canada, and Social Sciences and Humanities Research Council of Canada 2010). Chapter 6 of TCPS 2, "Governance of research ethics review," contains a section devoted to research ethics review during publicly declared emergencies[1]. As the TCPS is mainly geared towards "national" emergencies involving Canadian researchers, it puts the onus on the (academic) institutions to guarantee adequate ethics review, including greater-than-normal attention to risk. The main requirement is that institutions and their ethics review boards (ERBs) should develop preparedness plans for emergency research ethics review giving particular attention to timeliness of the process, availability of ERB members and coordination across institutions. The institution should also anticipate what research, if any, needs to be done during an emergency. The TCPS emphasises that exceptions to "normal" review procedures and infringement on ethical principles must be demonstrably justified.

[1] Defined in the TCPS 2 as '... extraordinary events that arise suddenly or unexpectedly, and require urgent or quick responses to minimize devastation. Examples include hurricanes and other natural disasters, large communicable disease outbreaks, catastrophic civil disorders, bio-hazardous releases, environmental disasters, and humanitarian emergencies. They tend to be time-limited. They may severely disrupt or may destroy normal functioning of institutions and communities, as well as individual lives' (2010, p. 85).

12.3.3 Working Group on Disaster Research and Ethics

Having witnessed violation of ethical norms in interventions and research carried out in the aftermath of the 2004 tsunami, Sri Lankan and international academics and researchers formed a group to counter the exploitation of vulnerable populations. The Working Group on Disaster Research and Ethics (WGDRE) was formed in 2007 and has produced a set of ethical guidelines applicable to post-disaster research with a developing world perspective (Sumathipala et al. 2010). These guidelines state that a stronger ethical obligation is required in disaster-related research and include eight specific recommendations concerning ethics review. Some specifically address the governance of ethics review:

- Independent, multidisciplinary and pluralist ethics committees should assess the research projects and include representation from the disaster-affected community
- Local ethics review is mandatory
- There should be a centralised mechanism for review and coordination of all research in the disaster-affected area to prevent unjustified repetitive work
- Prior ethics review and approval are possible, but research should start only after consultation with the actual disaster-affected community
- Expedited review is acceptable in exceptional situations with extreme caution and with quorum agreed beforehand.

These are the most detailed guidelines available to date which focus specifically on disaster-related research in developing country contexts.

12.3.4 A Framework for Ethics Review During Public Emergencies

Triggered by the outbreak of the H1N1 influenza pandemic in 2009, a group of Canadian researchers have proposed an alternative framework for research ethics review during emergencies (Tansey et al. 2011). Acknowledging the value of the TCPS 2, but also its shortcomings, they propose a more specific procedural framework based on the concepts of proportionate review, special scrutiny and expedited review. In their view, an explicit combination of these three elements could increase procedural flexibility and thus speed, while at the same time ensuring diligence proportionate to the risks and uncertainties involved. Figure 12.2 presents the main elements of the framework graphically.

The review process implies that the most intense scrutiny is for the most ethically challenging research. To ensure in-depth review more reviewers than usual would be assigned to protocols that are complex or pose high risk to participants or communities, but their assessment would be directed to specific aspects of the research. Other means to enhance diligence of the ERB would be frequent sequential reviews, increased monitoring, oversight of the informed consent process and additional expertise from non-ERB members to assess scientific validity and risks and benefits.

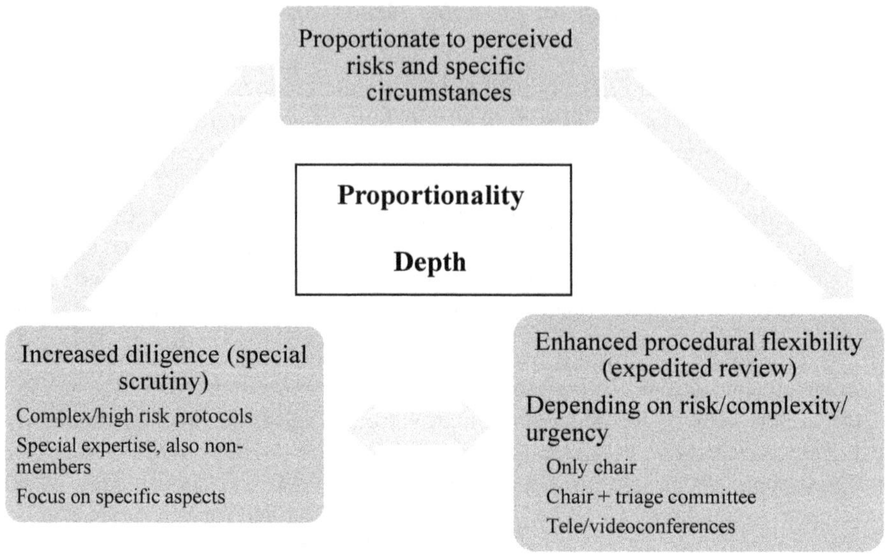

Fig. 12.2 A framework for ethics review during public emergencies. (Based on Tansey et al. 2011)

Expedited review by the chair would be acceptable only in cases of minimal risks. Tele/videoconferences are suggested as a way to overcome the difficulties of organising an ERB meeting at short notice. The authors suggest pilot-testing the proposed emergency procedures under "normal" circumstances.

While the CIOMS guidelines and the TCPS 2 mainly reaffirm the need to submit research carried out in emergency situations to ethical review, the WGDRE proposes more specific and detailed guidance for ethics governance with a particular focus on developing countries. Finally, the Canadian researchers develop a procedural framework with some very practical recommendations. However, their framework was developed in the context of a national public emergency in a highly resourced country with strong academic institutions. The next section will describe how some of the elements proposed by the WGDRE and the Canadian group have been tested by the ethics review board of one of the main international humanitarian aid organisations.

12.4 The Ethics Review Board of Médecins Sans Frontières

Médecins Sans Frontières (MSF) provides emergency medical assistance to populations in danger in more than 80 countries. In its work MSF is often confronted with situations for which effective and feasible interventions are lacking. In recent years MSF has expanded its research activities (Brown et al. 2008; Delisle et al. 2005; Pecoul et al. 1999; Trouiller et al. 2008). Although MSF often works in close collaboration with ministries of health and scientific institutions that have their own ethical review mechanisms, MSF as a humanitarian organisation has concerns that are distinct from academic institutions and wants to be confident in its endorsement of any research proposed to take place under its responsibility (Gilman and Garcia 2008; Nuffield Council on Bioethics 2002; Dieudonné 2007). Furthermore, not all countries in which MSF works have ethics committees or other means to oversee the ethics of research, and in some instances local ethics committees may not have the resources to function optimally (Elsayed and Kass 2007; Hyder et al. 2004; Ikingura et al. 2007; Kass et al. 2007; Rab et al. 2008). Furthermore, the local or national government is not always a guarantor for the wellbeing of the population MSF assists. For these reasons, MSF decided to institute its own ethics review board (MSF ERB) in 2001 (Schopper et al. 2009).

12.4.1 Functioning of the MSF ERB

Currently the MSF ERB has eight members with an understanding of humanitarian and NGO realities, ensuring geographic (Africa, Asia, Europe, North America) as well as professional (medicine, public health, law, sociology, bioethics) variety (Canadian Institutes of Health Research, Natural Sciences and Engineering Research Council of Canada, and Social Sciences and Humanities Research Council of Canada 2008; CIOMS 2009). To avoid conflict of interest and ensure independence, members cannot have a working relationship with MSF or be members of the board of an MSF entity during their tenure on the MSF ERB. Working procedures are defined in the terms of reference of the ERB (MSF 2009). Protocols are submitted by the MSF medical director responsible for the research. Reviews are coordinated by the chair of the ERB with comments being provided electronically. Discussions on divergent views take place mainly through e-mail exchange. Most frequently the reply by the researchers to the initial review of their proposal leads to a second round of questions and suggestions. In most instances, the second reply is satisfactory to allow approval. Thereafter it is the responsibility of the medical director to ensure that the research is implemented according to the ERB's remarks and approval. ERB members meet in person with the MSF medical directors every 18 months to discuss ethical issues that appeared as problematic in the reviews and make recommendations. These recommendations are binding, directly influence research practice and lead to the development of new standards and procedures.

12.4.2 A Framework with Benchmarks

During its first two years, the ERB used a framework derived from general guidelines on research ethics such as the Declaration of Helsinki (World Medical Association 2008), the Belmont Report (National Commission for the Protection of Human Subjects of Biomedical and Behavioral Research 1979) and the CIOMS guidelines

(CIOMS 2009). This provided a basis for discussion in case of diverging opinions. In 2003, in order to provide structured advice to field researchers and to facilitate standardised reviews, the ERB decided to adapt a draft framework for clinical research in the developing world developed by the National Institutes of Health in the United States (Emanuel et al. 2004). Its main advantages are that it is tailored for the developing world context and it sets practical benchmarks for each of the ethical principles. It does not add ethical requirements but makes them explicit and systematic. The framework was tested by the ERB over a period of 18 months to assess its utility and feasibility. As a result, some benchmarks were changed or expanded in three out of seven principles. Since March 2005, the revised version of the framework has been used (Ford et al. 2009). This framework has proven very valuable in standardising the review process, narrowing the scope of disagreement among ERB members and guiding field research teams in addressing ethical issues. Based on recent discussion, the framework is undergoing a further revision that will be submitted for final approval in September 2013.

12.4.3 Proportionality of Ethical Review

The MSF ERB recognises three types of ethical review, with different requirements. *Full review*, requiring participation of all ERB members, is warranted if a procedure or therapy of unknown effectiveness or efficacy is to be tested on human subjects or if the research involves collecting body or tissue samples for hypothesis testing (e.g. this covers all clinical trials and some operational research projects). *Expedited review*, requiring participation of two or three ERB members, is deemed sufficient if the research carries only minimal risks to human subjects. This includes descriptive studies involving monitoring and evaluation as a means to test a new approach, social science research in health and health systems, and studies of prevalence or incidence. Expedited review is proposed by the chair and can be challenged by the members. *Review exemption* applies to routine programme implementation, assessment related work and a posteriori analysis of routinely collected data. However, this last category only qualifies for review exemption if certain criteria are fulfilled: confidentiality is respected, no individual patient identifiers are revealed or used, and harm is null to minimal. In addition, there should be collaboration with a local authority or partner, and the research should have potential benefits to the community within which the research is being carried out. In case of doubt about the need for review, the medical director may submit the protocol for advice to the chair of the ERB. The stringency of the review process thus depends on the type of research.

12.4.4 Dealing with Emergency Research Ethics Review in MSF

In the past, MSF carried out research in emergency situations without requesting prior ethics review. This included nutrition and mortality surveys, probably of minimal risk to research participants, but also more complex studies such as testing a new treatment for acute malnutrition. The ERB was then asked to do an a posteriori review of emergency research when a report of that research was available as a draft paper, prior to submission to a scientific journal. This was deemed unacceptable and in June 2010 a procedure for ethics review of emergency research was agreed upon with the following elements:

- When researchers have decided what topic to research in the next emergency, a "generic" research protocol is submitted to the ERB for review and pre-approval before the exact location is known.
- Once the location is known, the final research protocol must be submitted to local ethics committee/authorities for approval.
- At the same time, the final proposal is submitted to the MSF ERB, including details pertinent to the chosen location. This review can be expedited by decision of the chair. This decision can, however, be challenged by one or more ERB members, leading to full ERB review.
- A posteriori ethics review by MSF ERB is no longer acceptable, but advice before publication can be provided.

This procedure had previously been tested in the case of a research protocol on meningitis treatment before an expected outbreak. The protocol was pre-approved for three countries, and the research was carried out in one of these countries.

As described above, some of the elements proposed in the procedural framework for ethics review during public emergencies (Tansey et al. 2011) are being implemented in practice by the MSF ERB, such as adapting the stringency of the review process to the potential risk of the research, functioning in a decentralised manner through electronic media, and using an expedited review mechanism. In addition, pre-approval of a "generic" research protocol, as proposed by the WGDRE, is a main element in the efforts to increase speed of the ethics review process when an emergency occurs, while at the same time ensuring diligence. None of the ethics governance mechanisms described in sect. 11.3 make reference to a pre-established ethics framework with specific benchmarks.

12.5 Ethical Issues Requiring Particular Vigilance

While ethics review of emergency and disaster-related research has to abide by the ethical principles governing all research on human subjects, some issues merit special attention. Some of these are addressed in more detail in other chapters of this book: harms and benefits to the disaster-stricken population (Chap. 8), informed consent (Chap. 9), and enhanced vulnerability (Chap. 11). Further issues that need special diligence on the part of ethics review committees in disaster/emergency situations are community involvement, dual use of tissue samples, and the humanitarian/therapeutic misconception. These will be described briefly in the next sections before drawing general conclusions and recommendations on research ethics governance.

12.5.1 Involving the Community

Frequently, disaster-related research is carried out in resource-constrained countries by Northern organisations. As highlighted by the WGDRE, researchers from "developed" countries may have little understanding of the local environment and their research agendas and interventions may act negatively on local vulnerable populations (Chap. 5; Sumathipala et al. 2010). The guidelines thus highlight the need for community participation before and during research in disaster-affected communities. However, this recommendation falls short of indicating how this can be done and what caveats might be needed. Defining who or what constitutes a "community" is particularly challenging in the humanitarian context where a community may be unstable and transient. Involving the "community" can also have negative consequences, if community leaders wield undue influence on potential research participants. Interfering with sound research procedures (sampling framework), inducing self-censorship due to political desirability and enforcing study participation have been highlighted as caveats of involving members of political and religious committees in research during war in Lebanon (Yamout and Jabbour 2010).

From an ethics perspective, community engagement should give the community a sense of ownership of the research, should ensure the relevance of the research and its cultural acceptability, should prevent exploitation and identify ethical hazards that may be part of the social, economic and political landscape of the community. Feedback to the community should be part of the community engagement process. An ERB should thus ensure that researchers enter into dialogue with the "right" community representatives, meaning those who truly represent the group in which the research will take place. These could be political representatives, leaders of local associations or any other person chosen as representative by a particular group. Collaboration with local researchers or consultation with government authorities does not equal community engagement.

12.5.2 Dual Use of Tissue Samples

Collection, exportation and analysis of tissue samples raise a host of ethical issues concerning the potential commodification and trafficking of human identity and the exploitation of communities from which tissues are taken. During emergencies, and in particular infectious disease outbreaks, samples are frequently sent from a developing country to a highly resourced country for diagnostic purposes. These samples may then be further used for research. For example, in the case of Ebola and Marburg haemorrhagic fevers, a limited number of reference facilities have a de facto monopoly on sample repositories and decisions on future use (Calain et al. 2009). Field reports attest to the fact that samples taken from patients for diagnostic purposes without explicit consent for research use, have then been used to test or develop new diagnostic procedures or therapies.[2]

Commentaries on Guideline 4, "Individual informed consent." of the CIOMS ethical guidelines, list a number of situations where it would be acceptable to waive consent in epidemiological surveillance studies. However, Guideline 24, "Use of stored biological samples and related data," makes it clear that secondary use of collected samples is only acceptable if informed consent was explicitly provided for future use (CIOMS 2009). Therefore, if samples are purposefully kept for future use, this should only be done with authorisation of the patient. The main issue is to respect the dignity of patients, making informed consent mandatory. In addition community engagement should be sought beyond individual-level consent (Upshur et al. 2007). In case of future use of anonymised individual samples at a time when contact has been lost with the patients, one needs to keep in mind that even if individual data are anonymised and thus harm to individuals is minimised, communities can be stigmatised by the publication of research results. Thus if individual consent can no longer be obtained for a posteriori use of tissue samples, at least community consent should be sought. Use of such samples would only be ethical if potential public health benefit clearly outweighs potential harms.

Even with consent, questions remain about the implications for individual patients and the community if research on these samples leads to commercial development of diagnostics, vaccines and treatments. This question of sharing potential benefits is essential, but well beyond the scope of this chapter.

12.5.3 The Humanitarian/Therapeutic Misconception

Most of the research carried out during or after disasters is not explicitly therapeutic in intent and will not directly benefit research participants. Potential research participants may be unaware of the difference between participating in a study and receiving clinical care as part of humanitarian aid, and are thus likely to misconceive research (interventions) as aid. In addition, some survivors may not anticipate that the research may induce distress by recalling emotionally painful memories (Collogan et al. 2004). The informed consent process must make the purpose of the research very clear and explicitly state that research is not part of clinical care. Researchers have a duty to ensure that potential study participants do not confuse research procedures with clinical care.

There may also be an unhealthy competition between public health practice and public health research in emergency situations. Disaster-stricken populations are very much in need of clinical and preventive public health services and research

[2] This issue has been highlighted by massive patent claims on antibodies and genes of bird flu survivors in September 2008. Samples from Vietnamese patients were taken in 2004 to the UK under a Wellcome Trust grant with "ethics approval". These samples were accessed by US and Swiss scientists and antibodies found to be highly effective against certain bird flu viruses. http://www.twnside.org.sg/title2/intellectual_property/info.service/2008/twn.ipr.info.081003.htm

should in no way interfere with the delivery of these services. But as repeatedly noted in the analysis of Ebola and Marburg fever outbreaks, the number of scientists studying the epidemic (epidemiologists, laboratory specialists, and field researchers) outnumbered experts providing patient care (Calain et al. 2009). If the normative principle that care has precedence over research is accepted, this implies a collective breach of duty to care. Research that can hinder rapid implementation of life-saving public health measures should be considered unethical. To prevent this, a standard of care below which patient care has *absolute* priority over research activities should be defined.

12.6 Conclusions and Recommendations

There is general agreement that research carried out in emergency and disaster situations must be submitted to ethical review and that the ethical obligation is stronger under such circumstances. But while there seems to be an increased awareness of the need to have clearer guidance for ethics review of such research, internationally accepted guidelines are lacking. Drawing on practical experiences, some researchers, groups and organisations have proposed ways to improve ethical oversight. The main elements to improve research ethics governance in disaster situations emerging from these proposals are:

12.6.1 Anticipate Emergency Research Before the Next Emergency

A "generic" research protocol should be designed prior to emergencies and submitted for provisional approval.

Potentially or previously affected communities should be involved ahead of time in the research development. This could, for example, be done in planning for research during epidemic outbreaks, through engagement with the Ministries of Health of countries with repeated outbreaks and involving potential victims or survivors in research development.

A pre-agreed upon framework for ethics review with defined benchmarks can ease the review process, allowing researchers to address issues at the initial stage of protocol development and streamlining the review by ERB members.

In instances where an international aid organisation anticipates research in a resource-constrained country, it should engage with and, if needed, strengthen local or national ethics review committees ahead of time

12.6.2 Timely, Flexible and Stringent Review when a Disaster Occurs

Timeliness and speed of the review procedure for (final) approval are enhanced through previous knowledge of the "generic" research protocol, electronic consultation among ERB members with additional telephone or videoconferencing if needed, and expedited review in case of minor changes to a pre-approved protocol or where there is judged to be minimal potential for harm to research participants. Expedited review is decided by the chair and includes at least one other ERB member. It can be challenged by any EBR member, leading to full ERB review.

In situations where local ethics review as well as review by the foreign (principal investigator's) institution is needed, dual review is mandatory (Ravinetto et al. 2010). The ERB of the foreign institution should include members having worked in emergency/disaster situations. If several national or international institutions are involved in the research, the need for multiple reviews by different ERBs should be questioned. The main question is how to avoid redundancy while respecting different institutional or national requirements. Delegation of ethics review responsibility to one national and one foreign ERB has been proposed. In this case, no more than two institutions should be in charge of the ethics review. Other review boards should be limited to registering and verifying the two ERB approvals (Gilman and Garcia 2008). Important research should not be delayed by increasing the bureaucracy of the review process (Collogan et al. 2004).

In case of a major disaster and many potential research activities and institutions, an oversight mechanism to prevent redundant research and oversampling of affected population must be put in place. How this could be done in situations where many organisations provide aid and the same or other institutions may engage in research activities, is still to be devised. ERBs can play an important role by at least demanding relevant information.

12.6.3 Some Issues Need Special Scrutiny

While the review procedure may vary depending on the type of research, three central questions have to be examined in every research endeavour in disaster situations.

- Is the research relevant to the population affected by the disaster or to populations in similar situations?
- Is the research feasible under prevailing circumstances in a disaster setting?
- Can the research question only be answered by carrying out research in a disaster-stricken population?

Only if the answer to all these questions is yes, should research be considered.

In addition ERBs should be particularly attentive to the issues descried in Sect. 11.5, namely:

- The boundaries between research and the delivery of a public health or medical intervention must be clearly defined and potential participants made well aware of the difference.
- Local community representatives must be involved, but this should not lead to undue influence on research participants.
- Tissue samples should be taken out of the country, or used for research purposes, only with explicit consent of patients.

In light of the deficit in international guidance about ethical oversight for emergency research, the fact that national regulations are frequently not adequate to govern ethical appraisal of research carried out in disaster-affected populations, and that such research activities are likely to increase in the coming years, an internationally recognized body should rapidly develop such guidance in collaboration with relevant organizations.

References

Brown, Vincent., Philippe J. Guerin, Dominique Legros, Christophe Paquet, Bernard Pécoul, and Alain Moren. 2008. Research in complex humanitarian emergencies: The Médecins Sans Frontières/Epicentre experience. *PLoS Medicine* 5: 553–556.

Calain, Philippe., Nathalie Fiore, Marc Poncin, and Samia A. Hurst. 2009. Research ethics and international epidemic response: The case of Ebola and Marburg hemorrhagic fevers. *Public Health Ethics* 2: 7–29.

Canadian Institutes of Health Research, Natural Sciences and Engineering Research Council of Canada, and Social Sciences and Humanities Research Council of Canada. 2008. Tri-Council Policy Statement: Ethical Conduct for Research Involving Humans.

Canadian Institutes of Health Research, Natural Sciences and Engineering Research Council of Canada, and Social Sciences and Humanities Research Council of Canada. 2010. Tri-Council Policy Statement: Ethical Conduct for Research Involving Humans.

Collogan, Lauren K., Farris Tuma, Regina Dolan-Sewell, Susan Borja, and Alan R. Fleischman. 2004. Ethical issues pertaining to research in the aftermath of disaster. *Journal of Traumatic Stress* 17: 363–372.

Council for International Organizations of Medical Sciences (CIOMS). 2002. *Ethics and research on human subjects. International ethical guidelines*. Geneva: CIOMS c/o WHO.

Council for International Organizations of Medical Sciences (CIOMS). 2009. *International Ethical Guidelines for Epidemiological Studies*. Geneva: CIOMS c/o WHO.

Delisle, Hélène., Janet Hatcher Roberts, Michelle Munro, Lori Jones, and Theresa W Gyorkos. 2005. The role of NGOs in global health research for development. *Health Research and Policy Systems* 3: 1–21.

Dieudonné, Désiré DA. 2007. Research ethics and developing countries. *Journal Inernational de Bioéthique* 18: 69–73.

Elsayed, Dya Eldin M., and Nancy E. Kass. 2007. Assessment of ethical review process in Sudan. *Developing World Bioethics* 7: 143–148.

Emanuel, Ezekiel J., David Wendler, Jack Killen, and Christine Grady. 2004. What makes clinical research in developing countries ethical? The benchmarks of ethical research. *Journal of Infectious Diseases* 189: 930–937.

Fleischman, Alan R., and Emily B. Wood. 2002. Ethical issues in research involving victims of terror. *Journal of Urban Health* 79: 315–321.

Ford, Nathan., Edward J Mills, Rony Zachariah, and Ross Upshur. 2009. Ethics of conducting research in conflict settings. *Conflict and Health* 3: 7.

Gilman, Robert H., and Hector H. Garcia. 2008. Ethics review procedures for research in developing countries: A basic presumption of guilt. *Canadian Medical Association Journal* 171: 248–249.

Halila, Ritva. 2007. Assessing the ethics of medical research in emergency settings: How do international regulations work in practice? *Social Science and Medicine* 13: 305–313.

Hyder, A.A., S.A. Wali, A.N. Khan, N.B. Teoh, N.E. Kass, and L. Dawson. 2004. Ethical review of health research: A perspective from developing country researchers. *Journal of Medical Ethics* 30: 68–72.

Ikingura, J.K., M. Kruger, and W. Zeleke. 2007. Health research ethics review and needs of institutional ethics committees in Tanzania. *Tanzania Health Research Bulletin* 9: 154–158.

Kass, Nancy E., Adnan Ali Hyder, Ademola Ajuwon, John Appiah-Poku, Nicola Barsdorf, Dya Eldin Elsayed, Mantoa Mokhachane, Bavon Mupenda, Paul Ndebele, Godwin Ndossi, Bornwell Sikateyo, Godfrey Tangwa, and Paulina Tindana. 2007. The structure and function of research ethics committees in Africa: A case study. *PLoS Medicine* 4: 26–31.

Leaning, Jennifer. 2001. Ethics of research in refugee populations. *Lancet* 357: 1432–1433.

Médecins, Sans Frontières. 2009. MSF field research: MSF ethics. http://fieldresearch.msf.org/msf/handle/10144/11645. Accessed 10 June 2013

National Commission for the Protection of Human Subjects of Biomedical and Behavioral Research. 1979. *The Belmont Report. Ethical Principles and Guidelines for the protection of human subjects of research*. Washington, D.C.: Department of Health, Education, and Welfare. National Instituters of Health.

Nuffield Council on Bioethics. 2002. *The ethics of research related to health care in developing countries*. London: Nuffield Council on Bioethics.

Oakes, J. Michael. 2002. Risks and wrongs in social science research: An evaluator's guide to the IRB. *Evaluation Review* 26: 443–479.

O'Mathúna, Dónal P. 2010. Conducting research in the aftermath of disasters: Ethical considerations. *Journal of Evidence Based Medicine* 3: 65–75.

Pecoul, Bernard., Pierre Chirac, Patrice Trouiller, Jacques Pinel, and Médecins Sans Frontières. 1999. Access to essential drugs in poor countries. A lost battle? *Journal of the American Medical Association* 281: 361–367.

Rab, Mohammad Abdur., Mohammad Afzal, Alaa Abou-Zeid, and Henry Silverman. 2008. Ethical practices for health research in the Eastern mediterranean region of the World Health Organization: A retrospective data analysis. *PLoS One* 3: 1–7.

Ravinetto, R., H. Tinto, N. Roumaba, A. Talisuna, Y. Adoke, A. Kadima Ebeja, V. Maketa, K.P. Grietens, A. Buvé, and F. Crawley. 2010. Health research: The challenges related to ethical review and informed consent in developing countries. *Giornale Italiano di Medicina Tropicale* 15: 15–20.

Schopper, Doris., Upshur Ross, Matthys Francine, Jerome Amir Singh, Sunita Sheel Bandewar, Aasim Ahmad, and Els van Dongen. 2009. Research ethics review in humanitarian contexts: The experience of the Ethics Review Board of Médecins Sans Frontières. *PLoS Medicine* 6: e1000115. doi:10.1371/journal.pmed.1000115.

Sumathipala, Athula., Aamir Jafarey, Leonardo D. de Castro, Aasim Ahmad, Darryl Marcer, Sandya Srinivasan, Nandini Kumar, Sisira Siribaddana, Sleman Sutaryo, Anant Bhan, Dananjaya Waidyaratne, Sriyakanthi Beneragama, Chandrani Jayasekera, Sarath Edirisingha, and Chesmal Siriwardhana. 2010. Ethical issues in post-disaster clinical interventions and research: A developing world perspective. Key findings from a drafting and consensus generation meeting of the Working Group on Disaster Research and Ethics (WGDRE) 2007. *Asian Bioethics Review* 2: 124–142.

Tansey, Catherine M., Margaret S. Herridge, Ronald J. Helsegrave, and James V. Lavery. 2011. A framework for ethics review during public emergencies. *Canadian Medical Association Journal* 182: 1533–1537.

Trouiller, Patrice., Piero Olliaro, Els Torreele, James Orbinsky, Richard Laing and Nathan Ford. 2008. Drug development for neglected diseases: a deficient market and a public-health failure. *Lancet* 359: 2188–2194.

Upshur, Ross EG., James V Lavery, and Paulina O. Tindana. 2007. Taking tissue seriously means taking communities seriously. *BMC Medical Ethics* 8: 1–6.

World Medical Association. 2008. World Medical Association Declaration of Helsinki: Ethical principles for medical research involving human subjects.

Yamout, R., and S. Jabbour. 2010. Complexities of research during war: Lessons from a survey conducted during the summer 2006 war in Lebanon. *Public Health Ethics* 3: 293–300.

Zwi, A.B., N.J. Grove, C. Mackenzie, E. Pittaway, D. Zion, D. Silove, and D. Tarantola. 2006. Placing ethics in the centre: Negotiating new spaces for ethical research in conflict situations. *Global Public Health* 1: 264–277.

Chapter 13
Ethical Concerns in Disaster Research—A South African Perspective

Keymanthri Moodley

13.1 Introduction

As a young democracy on the African continent, South Africa is home to approximately 50 million people from diverse cultural and religious backgrounds. Eleven official languages are recognised in celebration of the country's rich diversity. South Africa is a country of contrasts and paradoxes with a GINI coefficient of inequality of 0.72 indicating a wide divide between developed and developing world communities within the country (World Bank 2011). The GINI coefficient is the most commonly used measure of inequality and varies between zero (which reflects complete equality) and one (which reflects complete inequality). Private health care providers offer outstanding medical care to 20 % of the country's population while the public health care providers and institutions cater to the basic health care needs of 80 % of the population (Keeton 2010).

Geographically, the continent of Africa is generally stable and South Africa lies at its southern tip away from major tectonic plates. As such this region usually is not noted for any major natural disasters like earthquakes or tsunamis. In 1969 the strongest recorded earthquake in South Africa occurred in Ceres in the Western Cape. It scored 6.3 on the Richter scale. Thirteen people were killed and there was damage amounting to US$24 million (Wallis and Smith 2011). Between 1980 and 2010, 77 natural disasters occurred in which 1869 people lost their lives. During these three decades flooding occurred in 1987, 1994, 1981 and 2000 and accounted for 900 deaths. The remaining deaths were due to droughts and storms (Prevention Web 2011). In addition, thousands of others were injured and, if not physically harmed, suffered psychosocial trauma due to displacement and relocation. Many of these natural disasters occur in informal settlements and affect indigent populations who are doubly traumatised by these unforeseen events that are beyond their control. The devastating floods that occurred in 1994 in the Cape Flats prompted the government

K. Moodley (✉)
Stellenbosch University, Tygerberg, South Africa
e-mail: km@sun.ac.za

D. P. O'Mathúna et al. (eds.), *Disaster Bioethics: Normative Issues When Nothing is Normal,* Public Health Ethics Analysis 2, DOI 10.1007/978-94-007-3864-5_13,

to review civil protection in South Africa. In 1997 an Inter-Ministerial Committee for Disaster Management (IMC) was established (Wallis and Smith 2011).

With its history of apartheid under the rule of a white Afrikaner nationalist government from 1948 to 1994, South Africa had a tradition of discrimination that provoked political unrest. As such man-made disasters in the form of political unrest, riots, strikes and bombings were a frequent occurrence prior to democracy in 1994. Of note the Soweto riots in 1976 involved approximately 15,000 young people who marched in protest against being forced to learn Afrikaans—the language of their oppressor—in schools. Violent clashes with police resulted in thousands of injuries and approximately 172 deaths during one of the worst episodes of political unrest in the country (Mouton and Pohlandt-McCormick 1999). More recently, in 2008, South Africa experienced widespread outbreaks of xenophobic violence following the migration of people from African countries north of the country. Violent outbreaks started in Alexandra, an overcrowded informal settlement next to the affluent suburb of Sandton, Johannesburg. The violence quickly spread throughout the country (Kapp 2008). The attacks against foreigners claimed the lives of at least 62 people, 670 were injured, 1300 were arrested and 100,000 others were displaced throughout the country (Vromans et al. 2011). A significant volume of social science and mental health research followed in the wake of both these disastrous events.

13.2 A South African Disaster

Disasters are 'difficult to define with precision' (Rosenstein 2004, p. 373). In the usual sense of the word disasters are sudden, chaotic catastrophic events with an acute onset often resulting in significant physical, psychological, social and environmental harm. Loss of life and injury is usually of an extreme magnitude compared to morbidity and mortality in daily life. However a disaster may also be insidious in nature with a slow onset, escalating to a peak but leaving in its wake the same levels of physical and psychosocial harm as acute disasters. This is the typical morphology of epidemics and South Africa is no stranger to a host of infectious diseases that assume epidemic proportions on a regular basis.

In Africa outbreaks of meningococcal meningitis and viral haemorrhagic fevers have caused catastrophic loss of life over centuries. In South Africa the HIV/AIDS epidemic began with an insidious onset in the 1980s, but gradually came to a peak with massive loss of life over the next 30 years. Mortality reached its peak in 2000 with 600,000 or more deaths that year in South Africa alone. In the same year Kofi Annan remarked that HIV/AIDS had caused more loss of life in Africa than all the wars on the African continent (Brittain 2000). This comment was related to an HIV death rate of 6,000 Africans/day (UNAIDS 2010). In 2009 the number of HIV related deaths halved to 310,000. The total mortality since 1997 has been approximately 5 million. This is in stark contrast to the 1869 deaths attributable to natural disasters between 1980 and 2010.

In common with other types of disasters the HIV/AIDS public health disaster in South Africa has left people with acute and chronic sequelae. In particular the chronic impacts of 'social and economic hardship, loss of employment, the dissolution of personal relationships and the long-term deterioration of physical and mental health' are hallmarks of the aftermath of the HIV epidemic in this country (Collogan et al. 2004, p. 363). Approximately 15 million children under the age of 18 years have lost one or both parents due to AIDS. By 2008 there were approximately 1.4 million orphans in South Africa (WHO 2008). The phenomenon of child headed households is hence common-place. Stigmatisation of the disease has resulted in challenges with disclosure, testing and treatment. In some communities where disclosure has occurred in a hostile environment of stigma and shame, women have been killed by vigilante community members (Rossouw and Moodley 2011). Where HIV/AIDS is concerned, South Africa has operated in "disaster" mode for the past 30 years!

13.3 Disaster-related Research

Under these conditions it is important to study the clinical, psychosocial and environmental impacts on individuals, families and communities (Collogan et al. 2004). HIV/AIDS research has focused on treatment and prevention in adults, pregnant women and children, counselling, psychosocial support interventions, risks to health care workers, disclosure and stigma. Situated at the core of the epidemic in sub-Saharan Africa, South Africa presented an unparalleled opportunity for all kinds of research in the country. The past 30 years has seen an incremental growth in HIV research. Foreign funding and foreign researchers have steadily flowed into the country since the 1980s. Scientific, mental health and social science research has thrived. Approximately 1159 clinical trials are listed on the South African Clinical Trials Register. Of these at least 100 trials are related to HIV research. A host of ethical issues in the context of HIV research have emerged in South Africa especially in 1997 with the controversial vertical transmission trials (further details below).

Just as HIV research expanded, research into drug resistant tuberculosis (TB) has escalated. Two thousand new active cases of multi-drug resistant tuberculosis (MDR TB) occur each year in South Africa. Cure rates remain under 50 % and at least 30 % of cases are fatal within 2 years. Seventy percent of infections are chronic and infectious patients remain a threat to communities. It is predicted that there will be 2 million cases of MDR TB in South Africa by 2015 (Mazzotta 2010; Dheda et al. 2010).

13.4 South African Research Ethics Committees

Mindful of the growth of international collaborative research in the fields of HIV and TB and the need for dual review of research in both host and sponsor countries, local and national research ethics review capacity was accelerated. Although research ethics committees (RECs) had been in existence in South Africa since 1966 (Moodley and Myer 2007) the new public health disaster that started emerging in the 1980s and 1990s prompted RECs to consider their role in the assessment and approval of HIV related research—a field that promised to pose many new ethics review challenges for decades to come. The first national HIV vaccine workshop was held in 1998. The development of research ethics guidelines, structures and regulations progressed rapidly over the next three decades. In 1998, the Director-General of the Department of Health convened a working group to compile a national guideline for the conduct of clinical trials in South Africa. An Interim National Health Research Ethics Council (INHREC) was established in 2000. Guidelines for Good Practice in the conduct of clinical trials in human participants in South Africa were published in 2000 and are referred to as SAGCP. The purpose of the guideline was to provide South African researchers, RECs, research sponsors and the general public clearly articulated standards of good clinical practice in research that are contextualised to the local setting.

In 1997, at the height of the HIV/AIDS epidemic, South Africa had approximately 12 research ethics committees. By 2004 there were 22 RECs registered with INHREC and in 2011, there were 33 local RECs registered with a fully functioning National Health Research Ethics Council (NHREC). The second national research ethics guideline was released in 2004 by the Ministry of Health: *Ethics in Health Research: Principles, Structures and Processes*. Research that followed the onset of the HIV/AIDS public health disaster necessitated the development of a robust research ethics regulatory environment in the country. Such capacity development was accelerated by two large grants from the Fogarty International Centre of the National Institutes of Health. As a result, IRENSA (International Research Ethics Network in Southern Africa) and SARETI (South African Research Ethics Training Initiative) networks were established. In 2011 a new Fogarty funded program was established to replace IRENSA: Advancing Research Ethics training in Southern Africa (ARESA).

As a point of departure, it was important to ensure that "safari" or "parachute" research would not occur—a phenomenon which disaster research settings could lend themselves towards, where foreign researchers "parachute" in, conduct research and leave without local capacity development and without the research results impacting local communities (Siriwardhana 2007). In such settings those who bear the burdens of research do not benefit. Current national health research ethics guidelines specify that the health of South Africans must be improved by all types of research undertaken in this country. To ensure this, it was decided that all principal investigators should be either South African citizens or permanent residents in South Africa and that research should include provision for adequate capacity development.

The next important issue that was addressed was vulnerability. South Africa is home to millions of poor, disenfranchised communities subjugated during the apartheid era. These are communities that have been historically educationally disadvantaged and as a result there is inadequate understanding and experience with scientific and medical research. The Joint United Nations Program on HIV/AIDS

(UNAIDS) defines vulnerable communities as having some or all of the following characteristics:

1. Limited economic development
2. Inadequate human rights protection and discrimination based on health status
3. Inadequate community/cultural experience with the understanding of scientific research
4. Limited availability of healthcare and treatment options
5. Limited ability of individuals in the community to provide individual informed consent.

RECs and national research ethics guidelines routinely address vulnerability and the need for additional protections of such communities. In particular it is important to ensure that all consent information is presented in the relevant local languages using lay terminology. Respect for local customs, beliefs, culture and dignity is situated at the core of our national guidelines. In particular, community engagement and the formation of community advisory boards or groups is a prominent and central feature of most HIV research projects in South Africa.

13.5 South African Case Studies

13.5.1 HIV Prevention Trials in Pregnant Women

In 1997, at the height of the HIV/AIDS epidemic in South Africa, the standard of care debate emerged in the wake of HIV prevention trials on pregnant women in developing countries (Angell 1997; Coovadia and Rollins 1999; Moodley 1998). In 1994, the results of the first randomised placebo controlled study on pregnant women infected with HIV were published. It was established that treatment of these women with the antiretroviral drug zidovudine (or AZT) during pregnancy and delivery reduced the transmission of the virus from mother to child by 67 %. From this point onwards, zidovudine became the best proven standard of treatment for all HIV infected pregnant women in the United States (Connor et al. 1994).

The drug regimen used in this landmark study (called the ACTG 076 regimen) was, however, expensive and unaffordable in resource depleted countries. The next logical step was therefore to investigate the possibility of shorter and hence cheaper courses of treatment. UNAIDS and other organisations united to set up 16 clinical trials in 12 developing countries around the world. Nine of these studies were conducted by the National Institutes of Health (NIH) and the Centers for Disease Control and Prevention (CDC). One of these trials (conducted in Thailand) was designed as an equivalency study—three short course regimens were compared and the control group was given the ACTG 076 regimen. However, 15 of these 16 trials were randomised and placebo controlled. HIV infected pregnant women in the study group were given a short course of zidovudine and the incidence of transmission of the virus to their babies was established. However, the HIV infected pregnant women in the control group were given a placebo. And, this is where the controversy began.

In 1997, researchers with Health Research Group (an arm of the watchdog organisation, Public Citizen) drew attention to the ethical problems with such studies (Lurie and Wolfe 1997). They pointed out that all patients in similar studies in the US had unrestricted access to antiretroviral drugs unlike the 15 short course trials in developing countries which used placebos. An accompanying editorial written by the journal's executive editor, Marcia Angell, supported their views and compared these studies to the infamous Tuskegee syphilis study. This set in motion an unprecedented debate on the vertical transmission trials and the ethics of collaborative multinational research (Angell 1997).

Lurie and Wolfe argued that by conducting a placebo-controlled trial the researchers were, by implication, asking the wrong question: "Is the shorter regimen better than nothing?" The presumed answer to this question was that anything would be better than nothing. An essential pre-requisite to randomised clinical trials that compare two different treatments is that there should be no good reason to believe that one treatment is better than the other. This is called being in a state of clinical "equipoise." When there is clear evidence that one treatment is better than the other, 'not only would the trial be scientifically redundant, but the investigators would be guilty of knowingly giving inferior treatment to some participants in the trial' (Angell 1997, p. 847). During recruitment, researchers ask patients to submit to random assignment to one of two different treatments, one of which may be a placebo. This request can only be ethically justified if the researcher is in a state of genuine uncertainty regarding which treatment is better. This is so because randomisation is inconsistent with doing one's best for the patient as a doctor (Miller 2003). For intervention trials to be ethical, a potential new treatment should be compared with a placebo only when no known effective treatment exists. In the opinion of Lurie and Wolfe, the research question should have been: 'Can we reduce the duration of prophylactic [zidovudine] treatment without increasing the risk of perinatal transmission of HIV, that is, without compromising the demonstrated efficacy of the standard ACTG 076 [zidovudine] regimen?' (Lurie and Wolfe 1997, p. 855)

Defenders of the placebo trials argued in response that 'the most compelling reason to use a placebo-controlled study is that it provides definitive answers to questions about the safety and value of an intervention in the setting where the study is performed, and these answers are the point of the research' (Varmus 1997, p. 1003). This viewpoint was supported by a South African epidemiologist who argued that the fundamental research question related to whether short courses of antiretrovirals could reduce vertical transmission sufficiently to warrant their wide-scale implementation in South Africa (Abdool Karim 1998).

The investigators believed that it was not possible to extrapolate findings from the United States to Africa. The ACTG 076 regimen in the United States required that women receive HIV testing and counselling early in pregnancy, comply with oral treatment for several weeks, have intravenous antiretrovirals during labour and refrain from breast-feeding. In addition, babies would have to receive six weeks of oral antiretrovirals. South Africa, in common with other developing countries, has a high frequency of home deliveries especially in rural communities (Abdool Karim 1988). In developing country settings, women present late for antenatal care, have limited access to HIV testing and counselling and depend on breastfeeding to protect their babies from malnutrition and diarrhoeal diseases. The safety of zidovudine in populations who have a high incidence of malnutrition and anaemia was unknown. The cost of the ACTG 076 regimen was approximately $800 per treatment, far in excess of the per capita health care expenditure of under $10 in most developing countries (Varmus 1997). Charges were also made that criticism of the trials 'reflects a lack of understanding of the realities of health care in developing countries' (Halsey 1997, pp. 965–66). Many of these same arguments could be made about disaster research where the effectiveness of established interventions may be different in the midst of disaster conditions.

Others have objected to these trials based on the principle of justice. Annas and Grodin (1998) argued that poor participants should not bear the burdens of research that they would not benefit from. It was clear at the time the trials were conducted that the Ministry of Health in South Africa was not going to sanction the provision of short course antiretroviral treatment to pregnant women even if the trials did prove the treatment to be efficacious. This argument was underscored in Minister Zuma's decision in 1998 not to provide the four-week course of treatment to pregnant women (Knox 1998). In retrospect, that was probably a good decision. After all, the four-week treatment regimen did not prove to be efficacious (Petra Study Team 2002). However, the basic tenet of the argument remains valid—a protocol should contain a plan to implement efficacious results so that they benefit the research participants. This also applies to disasters where implementation of interventions as part of research in the acute phase should be made available to populations in the post-disaster phase.

13.5.2 HIV Vaccine Trials

Various other ethical issues have been raised by HIV research in South Africa. In particular HIV vaccine research has been fraught with scientific and ethical complexity (Moodley 2002). One of the earliest ethical dilemmas arose with respect to the clade (or viral subtype) that should be tested—the locally prevalent clade in South Africa (clade C) or clades that are prevalent in sponsor countries (such as clades A, B or E). At a meeting in 1998 it was decided by the Ministry of Health that a clade C vaccine should be tested in South Africa because if such a vaccine were found to be effective it would then benefit South Africans (Makgoba 1998). It was argued that South African communities should later benefit from bearing the burdens of research into a new vaccine. This was a very clear attempt to protect South African communities from exploitation where sponsors from developed countries would test a vaccine in South Africa that would never be useful for South African communities (because it was of the wrong clade type). This 1998 Ministry of Health ruling was later changed when scientists established that cross-clade reactivity might occur and hence other vaccine clades might also benefit South African populations (Moodley 2002).

Another ethical question is whether it is possible to obtain adequately informed consent from vulnerable participants who have difficulty understanding the scientifically complex issues inherent in vaccine trials. Educational thresholds of participants in high risk phase I trials created cause for concern as South Africa is home to many educationally disadvantaged populations. HIV vaccine trials are scientifically complex and many local South African languages do not have words to describe research and placebos amongst other terms. As a result, grade 12 education was set as a minimum requirement for participation in phase I HIV vaccine trials, and consent information and forms needed to be translated into local languages. Other matters of importance included the risk-benefit calculations necessary to review HIV vaccine trial protocols and access to treatment for participants who seroconvert during the course of the trials. Many of these issues are described and discussed in a national guideline produced by the Medical Research Council in South Africa (SAMRC 2003).

13.5.3 Co-enrolment and Co-infection Issues

Other HIV prevention trials have raised similar ethical issues—in particular microbicide research has been extremely challenging. Microbicide research had an unfortunate debut with early trials paradoxically demonstrating an increased risk of contracting HIV (Roddy et al. 1998; Van Damme et al. 2002). More recently, similar results have emerged with the premature closure of the cellulose sulphate trials at five developing country sites (Horwood 2007). South Africa has experienced co-enrolment on microbicide trials, high pregnancy rates on trials and challenges enrolling adolescents (Moodley 2007).

The alarming incidence of drug resistant tuberculosis in South Africa fuelled by the HIV epidemic has raised important scientific questions about treatment of the co-infection. Most recently, a study assessing different treatment regimens in patients co-infected with TB and HIV—the SAPIT trial— sparked an international bioethics debate on the vulnerability of research participants, clinical equipoise and the quality of research ethics review in South Africa (Abdool Karim et al. 2010). The SAPIT study investigated the timing of antiretroviral treatment (ART) in patients co-infected with TB and HIV. Patients were randomised to start ART in one of 3 phases of TB treatment: within 4 weeks of starting TB treatment, within 4 weeks of completing the intensive phase of TB treatment, or within 4 weeks of completing all TB treatment. Enrolment into the last group was stopped early by the Data Safety Monitoring Board (DSMB) due to higher mortality in this group. The higher death rates occurred in participants with a low CD4 count (less than 200). Critics have argued that the high mortality in participants with low CD4 counts could have been predicted and that these patients should not have been enrolled. They also argued that delaying ART until after TB treatment was below the standard of care (Boulle et al. 2010).

An influential editorial on the SAPIT trials entitled "A study that should not have been done" was a damning indictment of the researchers and the local ethics committee that approved the study (Philpott and Shuklenk 2010). The controversy has caused many scientists and ethicists globally to revisit the criteria for ethical research such as those concisely articulated by Emanuel and colleagues (2002).

13.6 Disaster Research Ethics

In response to the HIV/AIDS public health disaster, guideline development in South Africa is well advanced after 15–20 years addressing this situation. However, guidelines for disaster research more generally are not advanced, even though research frequently occurs during and in the aftermath of acute disasters. Several research studies followed the Soweto riots and the outbreaks of xenophobic violence in 2008 (Kapp 2008). These protocols were submitted to RECs in South Africa and were reviewed even though there are no specific guidelines for acute disaster research. While the national guideline deals with emergency research this refers to more everyday situations such as in the case of trauma research or ICU research. Here provision has been made for waiver of consent under very specific conditions. However research ethics review during acute disasters has not been specified in national guidelines.

When acute disasters strike, basic principles of health care ethics must be followed (Berg and King 2006). As a point of departure medical care and service delivery must take precedence over research in a resource depleted setting. The importance of prioritising clinical care during disasters is emphasised in the World Medical Association statement on Medical Ethics in the event of Disasters adopted in 1994 and revised in South Africa in 2006. According to this statement disasters create an 'unforeseen imbalance between the capacity and resources of the medical profession and the needs of survivors who are injured' and 'whose health is threatened' (WMA 2006, p. 1). Research in disaster settings is often conducted by people who are also involved in the provision of aid. As such research 'rightly takes second place to the provision of life-saving assistance' (Ford et al. 2009). A REC will therefore need to establish that care needs are met by medical personnel before such personnel will be permitted to conduct research in an acute disaster setting. In resource-depleted countries research will be viewed as a luxury during disasters (Siriwandana 2007).

In settings where medical care needs are met, the possibility of disaster research can be entertained provided that research can be conducted in a manner that is methodologically sound, practically feasible and ethically justified. Most research conducted during disasters involves descriptive or observational research—surveys, social science and mental health research (Wallis and Smith 2011). However the potential for ethical dilemmas exists with these types of research as well. REC members must weigh the societal benefits of disaster research against the individual risks to research participants.

Many have argued that research conducted during disasters in the acute setting has the potential to be beneficial in several ways (Collogan et al. 2004). In fact

Ford and colleagues argue that there is a 'clear justification and necessity to conduct research' during disasters (2009). Such research can help to report on the health and humanitarian consequences of disasters, to establish the prevalence of disaster related challenges and the types of health care services that are needed in different types of disasters. The most effective interventions with the lowest side effect profiles can also be established (Kilpatrick 2004). Models of healthcare delivery can be validated (Ford et al. 2009). However, benefits of research are inextricably linked to risk assessments.

While individual participants may benefit if the research interview is experienced as a form of catharsis and support (Newman and Kaloupek 2004), emotional harm may also result from revisiting traumatic experiences. 'A survey again? You are the third survey team who visited us during these couple of months. I am fed up with . . .' was the response that met researchers at the Zalingei Internally Displaced Persons camp in Darfur in 2004 (Aiga 2007, p. 823). Over-researching populations during acute disasters is an ethical concern. Between February and September 2004, 44 surveys were conducted in Darfur. Of 107 communities, 33 were subjected to two or more surveys and two communities underwent 5 or more surveys (Aiga 2007). Hence risks to participants must be assessed. This includes physical, psychological and social risks. Risks could include 'physical harm, inconvenience, legal action, economic hardship, psychological discomfort, loss of dignity, breach of confidentiality and unwanted media attention' (Collogan et al. 2004, p. 367). The level of REC review of research should be proportional to the risk associated with a specific project. This could range from expedited review of low risk research to full committee review for higher risk research. Full review of a generic protocol for anticipated projects that may occur in the setting of an acute disaster is also an option.

Once risk-benefit assessments have been completed, vulnerability and decisional capacity of potential participants are important considerations in resource-depleted settings. While one cannot assume vulnerability and impaired decision-making capacity in all settings of acute disasters (Levine 2004), many South African communities meet the UNAIDS criteria for "vulnerable communities". It has been argued that individuals under significant stress are able to make rational decisions about clinical care and research participation (Rosenstein 2004). However empirical research in South Africa (Abdool Karim 1998; Joubert 20033; Moodley et al. 2005) and in other parts of Africa (Molyneux et al. 2004; Frimpong-Mansoh 2008) has shown that under normal non-disaster circumstances, obtaining informed consent from study participants is challenging. Acute disasters add an additional layer of complexity and therefore decisional-capacity must be carefully assessed. Given the need for medical care in acute disasters, therapeutic misconception is likely to be highly prevalent and this should be actively guarded against in the consent process. Participants will need to be made aware that they are consenting to research only and that no expectations of care should be created. At the same time, should participants experience interviews as traumatic or emotionally distressing adequate provision should be made to arrange for counselling or debriefing. This must not be confused with therapeutic counselling services that may be on offer from other medical or mental health teams.

The principle of justice in research may be fulfilled by ensuring that those who carry the burdens of research stand to benefit. Despite almost 30 years of HIV research in South Africa only 50 % of patients who are eligible for treatment actually have access to treatment (UNAIDS Fact sheet). Of the 440,000 people with drug resistant TB less than 7 % are on treatment. A poignant question that must be raised in resource constrained settings is: "Do those who bear the burdens of research actually benefit?" Research protocols frequently postulate benefit to individuals and communities when attempting to justify projects. However after the research, many benefits do not materialise. Despite the post-research obligations specified in the Declaration of Helsinki (WMA 2008), participants in resource depleted settings often find themselves no better off when the research has ended. It is therefore crucial for any REC reviewing protocols for research during or after disasters to assess plans for post research benefit to communities. This should include a plan to return research results to participants anticipating that participants could be relocated in the months following the disaster

A robust research ethics regulatory environment has developed in South Africa because of its 30 years of experience addressing ethical concerns related to the public health disaster of HIV/AIDS. The emerging epidemic of drug-resistant tuberculosis brings with it some new challenges, but many areas are addressed in existing guidelines. The way forward now requires an emphasis on acute disaster research ethics formalised in national guidelines and in standard operating procedures of RECs. It behoves all researchers working in the field of mental health, environmental health and social science to anticipate future projects that may be significant in the face of an acute disaster and to start early protocol development. This must occur in parallel with REC consultations so that researchers are prepared when the next disaster occurs.

13.7 Conclusion

South Africa has a wealth of experience in addressing the scientific and ethical aspects of research during a chronic public health disaster, namely HIV/AIDS. Although less common, acute disasters in the form of political unrest, xenophobic violence and flooding do occur, yet RECs lack guidance for reviewing research conducted in such acute settings. Methodologically sound research conducted in acute disaster settings has the potential to yield valuable data. However in such settings research may be conducted by healthcare personnel who have assumed primary responsibility for care. RECs therefore have an obligation to ensure that healthcare needs are met first. If it is feasible to conduct sound research, RECs should conduct risk-benefit assessments of proposed research and ensure cultural and contextual appropriateness of consent processes given that South African populations often have enhanced vulnerability. Acute disasters create situations of instability and some populations may become inaccessible while others may be accessed more easily by research teams. Under these circumstances avoiding exploitation and over-researching of populations is critical.

In the recovery phase of acute disasters post-research obligations to populations must be honoured. The safe conduct of appropriate research during disasters (both acute and chronic) is an ethical imperative. Research that is conducted in acute disasters must be seen through to completion and publication is critical.

References

Abdool Karim, Quarraisha, Salim S. Abdool Karim, Hoosen M. Coovadia, and Merwyn Susser. 1988. Informed consent for HIV testing in a South African hospital: Is it truly informed and truly voluntary? *American Journal of Public Health* 88: 637–640.

Abdool Karim, Salim S., Kogieleum Naidoo, Anneke Grobler, Nesri Padayatchi, Cheryl Baxter, Andrew Gray, Tanuja Gengiah, Gonasagrie Nair, Sheila Bamber, Aarthi Singh, Munira Khan, Jacqueline Pienaar, Wafaa El-Sadr, Gerald Friedland and Quarraisha Abdool Karim. 2010. Timing of initiation of antiretroviral drugs during tuberculosis therapy. *New England Journal of Medicine* 362: 697–706.

Abdool Karim, Salim S. 1998. Placebo controls in HIV perinatal transmission trials: A South African's viewpoint. *American Journal of Public Health* 88: 564–566.

Aiga, Hirotsugu. 2007. Bombarding people with questions: A reconsideration of survey ethics. *Bulletin of the World Health Organisation* 85 (11): 823.

Angell, Marcia. 1997. The ethics of clinical research in the third world. *New England Journal of Medicine* 337: 847–849.

Annas, George., and Michael Grodin. 1998. Human rights and maternal-fetal HIV transmission prevention trials in Africa. *American Journal of Public Health* 88: 560–563.

Berg, Jessica., and Nicholas King. 2006. Strange bedfellows? Reflections on bioethics' role in disaster response planning. *American Journal of Bioethics* 6: 3–5.

Boulle, Andrew, Polly Claydon, Karen Cohen, Ted Cohen, Francesca Conradie, Krista Dong, Nathan Geffen, Ashraf Grimwood, Rocio Hurtado, Christopher Kenyon, Stephen Lawn, Gary Maartens, Graeme Meintjies, Marc Mendelson, Megan Murray, Molebogeng Rangaka, Iam Sanne, David Spencer, Jantjie Taljaard, Ebrahim Variava, W.D. Francois Venter, and Douglas Wilson. 2010. Prolonged deferral of antiretroviral therapy in the SAPIT trial: Did we need a clinical trial to tell us that this would increase mortality? *South African Medical Journal* 100: 566–571.

Brittain, Victoria. 2000. More die of Aids than war in Africa says Kofi Annan. The Guardian, March 14. http://www.guardian.co.uk/world/2000/mar/14/unitednations. Accessed 1 June 2013.

Collogan, Lauren K, Farris Tuma, Regina Dolan-Sewell, Susan Borja, and Alan R. Fleischman 2004. Ethical issues pertaining to research in the aftermath of disaster. *Journal of Traumatic Stress* 17: 363–372.

Collogan, Lauren K, Farris Tuma, and Alan R. Fleischman. 2004. Research with victims of disaster: Institutional review board considerations. *IRB: Ethics and Human Research* 26: 9–11.

Connor, Edward M., Rhoda S. Sperling, Richard Gelber, Pavel Kiselev, Gwendolyn Scott, Mary Jo O'Sullivan, Russell VanDyke, Mohammed Bey, William Shearer, Robert L. Jacobson, Eleanor Jimenez, Edward O'Neill, Brigitte Bazin, Jean-Francois Delfraissy, Mary Culnane, Robert Coombs, Mary Elkins, Jack Moye, Pamela Stratton, and James Balsley for the Pediatric AIDS Clinical Trials Group Protocol 076 Study Group. 1994. Reduction of maternal-infant transmission of human immunodeficiency virus type 1 with zidovudine treatment. *New England Journal of Medicine* 331: 1173–1180.

Coovadia, Hoosen M., and Nigel C. Rollins. 1999. Current controversies in the perinatal transmission of HIV in developing countries. *Seminars in Neonatology* 4: 193–200.

Dheda Keertan, Karen Shean, Alimuddin Zumba, Motasim Badri, Elizabeth Streicher, Liesl Page-Shipp, Paul Wilcox, Melanie-Anne John, Gary Reubenson, Darshini Govindasamy, Michelle

Wong, Xavier Padanilam, Alicia Dziwiecki, Paul D. van Helden, Sweetness Siwendu, Julie Jarand, Colin N. Menezes, Avril Burns, Thomas Victor, Robin Warren, Martin P. Grobusch, Martie van der Walt, and Charlotte Kvasnovsky. 2010. Early treatment outcomes and HIV status of patients with extensively drug-resistant tuberculosis in South Africa: A retrospective cohort study. *Lancet* 375: 1798–1807.

Emanuel, Ezekiel J., David Wendler, and Christine Grady. 2002 What makes clinical research ethical? *Journal of the American Medical Association* 283: 2701–2711.

Ford, Nathan, Edward J. Mills, Rony Zachariah, and Ross Upshur. 2009. Ethics of conducting research in conflict settings. *BMC Conflict and Health* 3: 7.

Frimpong-Mansoh, A. 2008. Culture and voluntary informed consent in African health care systems. *Developing World Bioethics* 8: 104–114.

Halsey, Neal A., Alfred Sommer, Donald A. Henderson, and Robert E. Black. 1997. Ethics and international research. *British Medical Journal* 315: 965–966.

Horwood, Jennifer. 2007. Cellulose sulphate microbicide trial halted. *Lancet Infectious Diseases* 7: 183.

Joubert, Gina, Hannes Steinberg, Elna van der Ryst, and Perpetual Chikobvu. 2003. Consent for participation in the Bloemfontein vitamin A trial: How informed and voluntary? *American Journal of Public Health* 93: 582–584.

Kapp, Clare. 2008. South Africa failing people displaced by xenophobia riots. *Lancet* 14: 1986–1987.

Keeton, Claire. 2010. Bridging the gap in South Africa. *Bulletin of the World Health Organisation* 88: 803–804.

Kilpatrick, Dean G. 2004. The ethics of disaster research: A special section. *Journal of Traumatic Stress* 17: 361–362.

Knox, Richard A. 1998. Despite epidemic, South Africa cuts AZT project. *Boston Globe Online*, December 1. http://www.aegis.org/DisplayContent/DisplayContent.aspx?sectionID=120031. Accessed 7 June 2013.

Levine, Carol. 2004. The concept of vulnerability in disaster research. *Journal of Traumatic Stress* 17: 395–402.

Lurie, P., and Sidney M. Wolfe. 1997. Unethical trials of interventions to reduce perinatal transmission of the human immunodeficiency virus in developing countries. *New England Journal of Medicine* 337: 853–855.

Makgoba, William. 1998. Should South Africa embark on clade B vaccine trials? Workshop on ethical issues in the conduct of HIV vaccine trials. Durban, South Africa.

Mazzotta, Meredith. 2010. HIV and drug-resistant tuberculosis in South Africa: A perfect storm. Science Speaks: HIV and TB News. http://sciencespeaksblog.org/2010/10/26/hiv-and-drug-resistant-tb-in-south-africa-a-perfect-storm/. Accessed 4 June 2011.

Miller, P. B., and C. Weijer. 2003. Rehabilitating equipoise. *Kennedy Institute of Ethics Journal* 13: 93–118.

Molyneux, C. S, N. Peshu, and K. Marsh. 2004. Understanding of informed consent in a low income setting: three case studies from the Kenyan coast. *Social Science and Medicine* 59: 2547–2560.

Moodley, Keymanthri. 1998. Preventing perinatal HIV transmission—does the end justify the means? *South African Medical Journal* 88: 809–810.

Moodley, Keymanthri. 2002. HIV vaccine trial participation in South Africa—An ethical assessment. *Journal of Medicine and Philosophy* 27: 197–215.

Moodley, Keymanthri, Michael Pather, and Landon Myer. 2005. Informed consent and participant perceptions of influenza vaccine trials in South Africa. *Journal of Medical Ethics* 31: 727–732.

Moodley, Keymanthri. 2007. Microbicide research in developing countries: have we given the ethical concerns due consideration? *BMC Medical Ethics* 8: 10.

Moodley, Keymanthri, and Landon Myer. 2007. Health research ethics committees in South Africa 12 years into democracy. *BMC Medical Ethics* 8: 1.

Mouton, Michelle, and Helena Pohlandt-McCormick. 1999. Boundary crossings: Oral history of Nazi Germany and apartheid South Africa—a comparative perspective. *History Workshop Journal* 48: 41–63.

Newman, Elana, and Danny G. Kaloupek. 2004. The risks and benefits of participating in trauma-focused research studies. *Journal of Traumatic Stress* 17: 383–394.

Petra Study Team. 2002. Efficacy of three short-course regimens of zidovudine and lamivudine in preventing early and late transmission of HIV 1 from mother to child in Tanzania, South Africa and Uganda (Petra study): A randomised double-blind, placebo-controlled trial. *Lancet* 359: 1178–1186.

Philpott, Sean, and Udo Schuklenk. 2010. A study that should not have been done. Bioethics Forum, May 5. http://www.thehastingscenter.org/Bioethicsforum/Post.aspx?id=4626&blogid=140. Accessed 1 June 2013.

Prevention Web http://www.preventionweb.net/english/countries/statistics/?cid=160. Accessed 2 June 2011.

Roddy, Ronald E, Léopold Zekeng, Kelley A. Ryan, Ubald Tamoufe, Sharon S. Weir, and Emelita L. Wong. 1998. A controlled trial of Nonoxynol 9 film to reduce male-to-female transmission of sexually transmitted diseases. *New England Journal of Medicine* 339: 504–510.

Rosenstein, Donald L. 2004. Decision-making capacity and disaster research. *Journal of Traumatic Stress* 17: 373–381.

Rossouw, Theresa, and Keymanthri Moodley. 2011. HIV/AIDS in South Africa: An exploration of the ethical options in Medical ethics, law and human rights: A South African perspective, ed. Keymanthri Moodley, 223–247. South Africa: Van Schaik.

South African Medical Research Council. 2003. Guidelines on ethics for medical research: HIV preventive vaccine research.

Siriwardhana, Chesmal. 2007. Disaster research ethics—A luxury or a necessity for developing countries. Asian Tribune.11: http://www.asiantribune.com/index.php?q=node/4524. Accessed 20 May 2011.

UNAIDS. 2010. *Global Report*. http://www.unaids.org/globalreport. Accessed 7 June 2013.

Varmus, H., and D. Satcher. 1997. Ethical complexities of conducting research in developing countries. *New England Journal of Medicine* 337: 1003–1006.

Van Damme, Lut, Gita Ramjee, Michel Alary, Bea Vuylsteke, Verapol Chandeying, Helen Rees, Pachara Sirivongrangson, Leonard Mukenge Tshibaka, Virginie Ettiegne-Traore, Charn Uaheowitchai, Salim S. Abdool Karim, Benoit Masse, Jos Perriens, and Marie Laga. 2002. Effectiveness of COL-1492, a nonoxynol-9 vaginal gel, on HIV-1 transmission in female sex workers: a randomized controlled trial. *Lancet* 360: 971–977.

Vromans, Lyn, Robert D. Schweitzer, Katharine Knoetze, and Ashraf Kagee. 2011. The experience of xenophobia in South Africa. *American Journal of Orthopsychiatry* 81: 90–93.

Wallis, Lee and Wayne Smith. 2011. Disaster Medicine. South Africa: Juta.

World Bank. 2011. Poverty analysis—Measuring inequality. http://go.worldbank.org/3SLYUTVYOO. Accessed 20 May 2011.

World Medical Association (WMA). 2006. Statement on medical ethics in the event of disasters. http:www.wma.net/en/30publications/10policies/d7/. Accessed 11 November 2011.

World Medical Association (WMA). 2008. Declaration of Helsinki: Ethical principles for medical research involving human subjects (revised). Geneva, Switzerland: World Medical Association. http://www.wma.net/en/30publications/10policies/b3/17c.pdf. Accessed 20 May 2011.

World Health Organisation (WMA). 2008. Epidemiological Fact Sheets: South Africa, 2008 Update. http://apps.who.int/globalatlas/predefinedReports/EFS2008/full/EFS2008_ZA.pdf. Accessed 30 May 2011.

Appendix I—Code of Conduct for the International Red Cross and Red Crescent Movement and NGOs in Disaster Relief

Purpose This Code of Conduct seeks to guard our standards of behaviour. It is not about operational details, such as how one should calculate food rations or set up a refugee camp. Rather, it seeks to maintain the high standards of independence, effectiveness and impact to which disaster response NGOs and the International Red Cross and Red Crescent Movement aspires. It is a voluntary code, enforced by the will of each organization accepting it to maintain the standards laid down in the Code.

In the event of armed conflict, the present Code of Conduct will be interpreted and applied in conformity with international humanitarian law.

Disasters A disaster is a calamitous event resulting in loss of life, great human suffering and distress, and large scale material damage.

Principles of Conduct for the International Red Cross and Red Crescent Movement and NGOs in Disaster Response Programmes

1. The humanitarian imperative comes first.
2. Aid is given regardless of the race, creed or nationality of the recipients and without adverse distinction of any kind. Aid priorities are calculated on the basis of need alone.
3. Aid will not be used to further a particular political or religious standpoint.
4. We shall endeavour not to act as instruments of government foreign policy.
5. We shall respect culture and custom.
6. We shall attempt to build disaster response on local capacities.
7. Ways shall be found to involve programme beneficiaries in the management of relief aid.
8. Relief aid must strive to reduce future vulnerabilities to disaster as well as meeting basic needs.

D. P. O'Mathúna et al. (eds.), *Disaster Bioethics: Normative Issues When Nothing is Normal,* Public Health Ethics Analysis 2, DOI 10.1007/978-94-007-3864-5,

9. We hold ourselves accountable to both those we seek to assist and those from whom we accept resources.
10. In our information, publicity and advertizing activities, we shall recognize disaster victims as dignified human beings, not hopeless objects.

Reproduced here with permission from the International Committee of the Red Cross (ICRC). The Code was prepared jointly by the International Federation of Red Cross and Red Crescent Societies and the ICRC. 29-02-1996 Article, International Review of the Red Cross, No. 310. Available with interpretive comments at http://www.icrc.org/eng/resources/documents/misc/code-of-conduct-290296.htm.

Appendix II—WMA Statement on Medical Ethics in the Event of Disasters

Adopted by the 46th WMA General Assembly, Stockholm, Sweden, September 1994 and revised by the 57th WMA General Assembly, Pilanesberg, South Africa, October 2006.

1. The definition of a disaster for the purpose of this document focuses particularly on the medical aspects.

A disaster is the sudden occurrence of a calamitous, usually violent, event resulting in substantial material damage, considerable displacement of people, a large number of victims and/or significant social disruption. This definition excludes situations arising from conflicts and wars, whether international or internal, which give rise to other problems in addition to those considered in this paper. From the medical standpoint, disaster situations are characterized by an acute and unforeseen imbalance between the capacity and resources of the medical profession and the needs of survivors who are injured whose health is threatened, over a given period of time.

2. Disasters, irrespective of cause, share several features:
   a. their sudden and unexpected occurrence, demanding prompt action;
   b. material or natural damage making access to the survivors difficult and/or dangerous;
   c. adverse effects on health due to pollution, and the risks of epidemics, and emotional and psychological factors;
   d. a context of insecurity requiring police or military measures to maintain order;
   e. media coverage.

Disasters require multifaceted responses involving many different types of relief ranging from transportation and food supplies to medical services. Physicians are likely to be part of coordinated operations involving other responders such as law enforcement personnel. These operations require an effective and centralized authority to coordinate public and private efforts. Rescue workers and physicians are confronted with an exceptional situation in which their normal professional ethics must be brought to the situation to ensure that the treatment of disaster survivors

D. P. O'Mathúna et al. (eds.), *Disaster Bioethics: Normative Issues When Nothing is Normal,* Public Health Ethics Analysis 2, DOI 10.1007/978-94-007-3864-5,

conforms to basic ethical tenets and is not influenced by other motivations. Ethical rules defined and taught beforehand should complement the individual ethics of physicians.

Inadequate and/or disrupted medical resources on site and the large number of people injured in a short time present specific ethical challenges.

The World Medical Association therefore recommends the following ethical principles and procedures with regard to the physician's role in disaster situations.

3. Triage
   1. Triage is a medical action of prioritizing treatment and management based on a rapid diagnosis and prognosis for each patient. Triage must be carried out systematically, taking into account the medical needs, medical intervention capabilities and available resources. Vital acts of reanimation may have to be carried out at the same time as triage. Triage may pose an ethical problem owing to the limited treatment resources immediately available in relation to the large number of injured persons in varying states of health.
   2. Ideally, triage should be entrusted to authorized, experienced physicians or to physician teams, assisted by a competent staff.
   3. The physician should separate patients into categories and then treat them in the following order, subject to national guidelines:
      a. patients who can be saved but whose lives are in immediate danger should be given treatment straight away or as a matter of priority within the next few hours;
      b. patients whose lives are not in immediate danger and who are in need of urgent but not immediate medical care should be treated next;
      c. injured persons requiring only minor treatment can be treated later or by relief workers;
      d. psychologically traumatized individuals who do not require treatment for bodily harm but might need reassurance or sedation if acutely disturbed;
      e. patients whose condition exceeds the available therapeutic resources, who suffer from extremely severe injuries such as irradiation or burns to such an extent and degree that they cannot be saved in the specific circumstances of time and place, or complex surgical cases requiring a particularly delicate operation which would take too long, thereby obliging the physician to make a choice between them and other patients. Such patients may be classified as "beyond emergency care".
      f. Since cases may evolve and thus change category, it is essential that the situation be regularly reassessed by the official in charge of the triage.
   4. The following statements apply to treatment beyond emergency care
      a. It is ethical for a physician not to persist, at all costs, in treating individuals "beyond emergency care", thereby wasting scarce resources needed elsewhere. The decision not to treat an injured person on account of priorities dictated by the disaster situation cannot be considered a failure to come to the assistance of a person in mortal danger. It is justified when it is intended to save the maximum number of individuals. However, the physician must

show such patients compassion and respect for their dignity, for example by separating them from others and administering appropriate pain relief and sedatives.

b. The physician must act according to the needs of patients and the resources available. He/she should attempt to set an order of priorities for treatment that will save the greatest number of lives and restrict morbidity to a minimum.

4. Relations with the patients
   1. In selecting the patients who may be saved, the physician should consider only their medical status, and should exclude any other consideration based on non-medical criteria.
   2. Survivors of a disaster are entitled to the same respect as other patients, and the most appropriate treatment available should be administered with the patient's consent. However, it should be recognized that in a disaster response there may not be enough time for informed consent to be a realistic possibility.
5. Aftermath of disaster
   1. In the post-disaster period the needs of survivors must be considered. Many may have lost family members and may be suffering psychological distress. The dignity of survivors and their families must be respected.
   2. The physician must respect the customs, rites and religions of the patients and act in all impartiality.
   3. If possible, the difficulties encountered and the identification of the patients should be reported for medical follow-up.
6. Media and other third parties
   The physician has a duty to each patient to exercise discretion and ensure confidentiality when dealing with third parties, and to exercise caution and objectivity and act with dignity with respect to the emotional and political atmosphere surrounding disaster situations. This implies that physicians are empowered to restrict the entrance of reporters to the medical premises. Media relations should always be handled by appropriately trained personnel.
7. Duties of paramedical personnel
   The ethical principles that apply to physicians also apply to personnel under the physician's direction.
8. Training
   The World Medical Association recommends that disaster medicine training be included in the curricula of university and post-graduate courses in medicine.
9. Responsibility
   The World Medical Association calls upon governments and insurance companies to cover both civil liability and any personal damages to which physicians might be subject when working in disaster or emergency situations.
   The WMA requests that governments:
   a. accept the presence of foreign physicians and, where demonstrably qualified, their participation, without discrimination on the basis of factors such as affiliation (e.g. Red Cross, Red Crescent, ICRC, and other qualified organizations), race, or religion.
   b. give priority to the rendering of medical services over visits of dignitaries.

Index

A
Abdool Karim, S.S., 196–198, 200
Accountability for reasonableness, 144
  concept of, 145
  limitations of, 145
Acute disaster, 200, 201
Agamben, G., 24
Ahmad, A., 67, 103
Aiga, H., 200
Alexander, D.A., 6
All-hazards preparedness doctrine, 139
Altevogt, B.M., 104
American culture, 125
Amputation, 30, 161
  clinical trials of, 139
Anand, S., 143
Anderson, E.D., 58
Anderson-Shaw, L., 15
Anecdotal evidence, 33
  literature and resources in, 34
Angell, M., 195, 196
Annas, G., 197
Annas, G.J., 104, 124, 129, 132, 136, 137, 139
Anthrax attack, 78, 166
Anticipatory review *See* Preapproved protocol, 138
Antiretroviral treatment (ART), 198
Apartheid, 194
  history of, 192
Appelbaum, P.S., 165
Assurance, 133, 144
AZT *See* Zidovudine, 195

B
Bagozzin, R.P., 46
Balicer, R.D., 85
Barilan, Y.M., 54
Barnett, B., 83
Barnett, D.J., 15, 86
Barnett, M., 21, 23, 28
Barzilay, E., 109
Beecher, H.K., 133
Belmont report, 181
Beneficence, 22, 59, 114
Benhabib, S., 23
Berg, J., 17, 199
Bhopal chemical explosion, 171
Bhugra, D., 66
Biafra war, 23
Big Tent research, 112
Biodefense, 29
Bioterrorism, 16, 29
Blackburn, S., 39
Blood draw, 168
Bobbitt, P., 53
Bohannon, J., 110
Boulle, A., 198
Boylan, J.F., 112
Bradt, D.A., 96, 97, 99–102
Brauman, R., 23, 30
Brittain, V., 192
Brown, C., 26, 27
Brown, V., 180
Buddhism, 66
Burial ritual, 66, 73
Burn-out, 8
  of healthcare professionals, 35
Burris, D.G., 49
Byerly, C.R., 89

C
Calabresi, G., 53
Calain, P., 168, 169, 175, 177, 184, 186
Call centre, 80, 83, 91
Camacho-McAdoo, G., 24
Capacity, 4, 23, 52, 57, 74, 96, 162, 164
Capacity building, 151

D. P. O'Mathúna et al. (eds.), *Disaster Bioethics: Normative Issues When Nothing is Normal,* Public Health Ethics Analysis 2, DOI 10.1007/978-94-007-3864-5,

Capacity development, 194
Capecitabine, 147
Carter, R., 137
Catholic, 72
Centre for Research on the Epidemiology of Disasters (CRED), 95
Charvet, J., 23
Chatterdjee, D.K., 22
Chernobyl nuclear accident, 160, 166, 171, 176
Children, 42, 55, 57, 72, 73, 77, 96, 109, 131, 164
  HIV/AIDS research in, 193
  research on, 119, 132
  studies on, 137
Chile 2010 earthquake, 19, 95
Cholera, 176
  epidemic of, 113
  prevention of, 36
  vaccination of, 72
Christie, T., 26
Citraningtyas, T., 66
Civil defence
  practice of, 16
Clark, N., 18
Clarke, M., 97, 100
Clinical equipoise, 162, 163, 198
Co-enrolment, 198
Coady, C.A.J., 27
Coercion, 163
Cognitive behavioural therapy (CBT), 101
Collins, F.S., 132
Collogan, L.K., 139, 185, 187, 193, 199, 200
Colonialism, 19, 34
Communication, 8, 51, 77, 80, 81, 88, 91
  guidelines on, 90
  in a health emergency, 78
  problems in, 91
  strategies of, 79
  training on, 83
  types of, 90
Community involvement, 65, 183
Compassion, 7, 22, 24–26, 28–30
Complete duty, 58
Complex emergency, 4, 18, 42, 95, 119
Confidentiality, 182
  breach of, 200
Conflict of interest, 67, 181
Connor, E.M., 195
Contract research organisations, 137
Conventional triage, 51
Coovadia, H.M., 195
Cosgrave, J., 101
Costello, A., 33
Council for International Organizations of Medical Sciences (CIOMS), 41, 117
  guidelines of, 120, 121, 163, 164, 178, 180, 181, 185
  International Ethical Guidelines for Biomedical Research, 117, 163, 178
  International Ethical Guidelines for Epidemiological Studies, 170
Cowan, E., 170
Credibility, 79, 81, 82, 84
Cremation, 66, 80
Crush injuries, 160–162
Culshaw, C., 151
Cultural difference, 8, 35, 79
Culture, 8, 46, 66, 67, 71, 195
  definition of, 66
  perspectives of, 66
  role of language in, 66
  role of religion in, 67
Cutler, J.C., 132
Cutler, John C., 131–133, 136
  syphilis studies by, 134

D

Daniels, N., 144, 145
Daniels, Norman, 144
Darfur, 200
  women of, 113
Data safety monitoring board (DSMB), 198
De Ville de Goyet, C., 30
de Waal, A., 36, 43
Dean, R.A., 165
Death, 26, 36, 45, 51, 52, 54, 61, 65, 66, 72, 80, 96, 162, 192
Debriefing, 71, 200
Debrix, F., 25
Deception, 132
Decisional-capacity, 200
Declaration of Helsinki, 114, 116, 117, 119, 163, 181, 201
Dehner, G., 78, 84
Delisle, H., 180
Democratic Republic of Congo, 27
Development, 10, 19, 20, 28, 43, 44, 96, 104, 181
  policies on, 153
  programme on, 151
Dheda, K., 193
Diamond, W., 96
Dieudonné, D.D.A., 181
Dignity, 7, 73, 123, 195
Disability, 49, 52, 54, 115, 146, 162, 166
Disaster, 10, 16, 19, 22, 37, 42, 53, 61, 95, 109, 132, 164

aftermath of, 101, 122, 171
aspects of, 113
categories of, 4
consequences of, 65, 122, 161, 200
definition of, 4, 17
ethical issues in, 7
impact of, 113
issues of, 4
research on, 159
types of, 8, 10, 17, 109, 170, 193
Disaster bioethics, 4–6, 42
macro-ethical perspective of, 7
Disaster care, 54, 56, 57
Disaster caretakers, 55
Disaster conditions, 37, 119, 120, 124, 125
research in, 118
Disaster ethics, 39
Disaster management, 99, 151
Disaster medicine, 53
Disaster planning, 13, 16, 103
analyses of, 29
Disaster relief, 6, 14, 15, 100
ethical framework of, 29
ethical problems in, 13
Disaster relief operations, 99, 100
Disaster relief response, 35
Disaster research, 6, 8, 91, 102, 110–112, 125, 138, 165, 176, 197, 199
ethical issues in, 6
Disaster research priorities, 143, 144, 147, 149, 150, 152–154
Disaster response, 6, 8, 38, 39, 99, 101
Disaster response planning, 17
Disaster risk reduction, 4
Disaster victims, 120, 121, 123, 125, 133, 135, 165, 166
research on, 129
Disaster's 6 Ds, 66, 67, 96
Disaster-affected communities, 65
Disaster-related research, 184, 193
Disaster-relief organizations, 86
Disasters, 30, 33–35
ethical issues in, 4
research ethics in, 139
Displaced persons, 96, 164, 171
Disruptive disaster, 51
Donors, 5, 37, 38, 41
Double disaster, 8, 51, 52, 58
Drug resistant tuberculosis (TB), 10, 193, 198
Dual use, 10, 169, 183, 184
Duty of care, 43, 45
DuVal, G., 33
Dynes, R., 86

E
Earthquake-tsunami disaster, 2011, 124
Ebola virus, 169, 176, 184, 186
Eddleston, M., 68
Edison, N., 83
Effective communication, 79
principles of, 77, 79
Ekanayake, S., 72
Elliot, A.J., 152
Elsayed, D.E.M., 181
Emanuel, E., 113
Emanuel, E.J., 111, 121, 123, 138, 182, 199
Emergency ethics, 23, 28–30
Emergency Events Database (EM-DAT), 95
Emergency medicine, 15
Emergency research, 129, 176, 178, 183, 188, 199
Emergency response, 170, 171
Emergency training exercise, 83
Empathy, 8, 79, 81
Enhanced Learning and Research for Humanitarian Assistance (EHLRA), 148
Environmental hazards, 151
Epidemiology, 71, 72, 97
Epstein, M., 112
Ethical hazards, 184
Etienne, M., 21, 33
European Convention on Human Rights and Biomedicine, 115
Euthanasia, 111
Eva, J., 5
Evidence, 8, 9, 41, 84, 91, 96–103, 146, 151, 165
definition of, 97
Evidence-based medicine (EBM), 96, 97
Eyal, N., 5
Eye Movement Desensitisation and Reprocessing (EMDR), 71

F
Facebook, 84
Fairchild, A., 168
Faith, 72, 115
False alarm, 84
Farmer, P., 109, 124, 138, 139
Farmer, Paul, 109, 124, 138
Fassin, D., 22–25
Fassin, Didier, 24
Federal Emergency Management Agency (FEMA), 16
Fernando, A.G., 71
Fiduciary commitments, 53
Fiduciary duties, 56, 58

Fiduciary relationship, 120
Financial capacity, 165
Fink, S., 111
Fire-fighter, 53, 90, 166
First come, first served, 55
Firth, P., 5
Fitzgerald, F.S., 125
Fixation surgery, 161, 162
Fleck, L., 53
Fleischman, A.R., 160, 171, 172, 176
Flynn, S., 30
Focus group, 112
Ford, N., 28, 176, 182, 199, 200
Foreign policy, 21, 29
Fost, N., 129
Fox, E., 33
Frieden, T.R., 132
Frimpong-Mansoh, A., 200
Fukushima Daiichi nuclear plant, Japan, 160, 166
Fuller, L., 27
Funes, J.M., 132

G

Gale, K.L., 82
Ganeshan, S., 96
Garcia, H.H., 181, 187
Garrett, L., 29
Gatrad, A.R., 66
Gender, 101, 146, 149, 161
Generalisable knowledge, 169
Gibson, J., 145
Gilbert, J., 66, 67
Gilman, R.H., 181, 187
GINI coefficient, 191
Glantz, L.H., 136
Glickman, S.W., 137
Globalisation, 22, 138
Good samaritan, 23
Grading of Recommendations Assessment, Development and Evaluation (GRADE), 98, 99
Graniger, S., 130
Greater good, 36
Greenhalgh, T., 97
Grodin, M., 197
Grodin, M.A., 132
Gross, M., 50, 51, 53
Grounded theory, 34
Gruskin, S., 144
Guantanamo Bay, 23
Guatemala, 130, 137
  STD experiments in, 131
  US medical research in, 9, 130
Guatemala experiments, 130–133, 136
Guatemala studies, 132, 133, 135, 136
Guyatt, G.H., 98, 99

H

H1N1 2009 influenza pandemic, 78, 84, 166, 179
Haiti 2010 earthquake, 3, 19, 20, 65, 167, 176
Hakan, A.K., 5
Halila, R., 177
Halsey, N.A., 197
Harm-benefit assessment, 111, 118–120, 122
Harm/benefit ratio, 111
Harman, G., 66
Hattori, T., 21, 22
Hazard, 150
  assessment of, 150
Health hazards, 111
Health inequalities, 146
Health Protection Agency (HPA), 148, 151
Heat wave, 3, 65, 95, 151
Herkert, J.R., 14
HIV 076 studies, 136, 137
HIV vaccine, 194
  research on, 197
  trials on, 198
HIV/AIDS, 10, 201
  in South Africa, 192
  pandemic of, 26
  research on, 193, 194
  studies on, 136
Hodge, J.G., 16, 58
Holm, S., 121
Hornblum, A.M., 122, 137
Horwood, J., 198
Hughes, D.A., 146
Human dignity, 11, 22, 26, 28, 58, 116, 130, 139
  notion of, 28
Human radiation experiments, 119, 131, 138
Human rights, 7, 9, 13, 15, 22, 28, 29, 124, 130, 139
  norms of, 22
  violations of, 23
Humanitarian aid, 7, 14, 18, 21, 22, 29, 30, 38, 43, 44, 67, 73, 152, 185
Humanitarian assistance, 21
Humanitarian disasters, 18, 50
Humanitarian health care
  ethics of, 34, 36, 37, 41
  practice of, 45–47
  providers of, 33, 34, 42

Humanitarian Health Ethics Analysis Tool (HHEAT), 44, 46
Humanitarian intervention, 22, 24, 27
Humanitarianism, 7, 13, 21, 23–28
Humanity, 21, 22, 24, 25, 150
Hunt, M.R., 39, 44, 47
Hurrell, C., 83
Hurricane Katrina, 3, 19, 26, 65, 96, 111, 164, 167, 176
Hyder, A.A., 181
Hyogo Framework for Action (HFA), 6

I
Ideal and non-ideal moral theory, 42
Iezzoni, L., 89
Ikingura J.K., 181
Impartiality, 21, 23, 24, 148
Incomplete duty, 58
Independence, 19, 21, 56, 146, 181
Indian Ocean 2004 tsunami, 3, 7, 18, 80, 101, 102
Individuals' capacity, 165
Inducement for research, 73, 103
Inequality, 24, 25, 191
Influenza epidemic, 166
Influenza pandemic of 1918, 80, 83
Informed consent, 9, 111, 112, 115, 119–123, 130, 132, 136–139, 152, 159, 162, 163, 165, 170, 171, 179, 185, 198, 200
  for patients, 41
  for research, 102
  importance of, 133
  in medical research, 116
  issues of, 7
  research on, 123
Injustice, 34, 36, 38, 39, 42, 43
Insidious, 192
Institutional review board (IRB), 114, 117
Integrated Research on Disaster Reduction (IRDR), 150
Internally displaced persons, 113, 200
International Committee of the Red Cross (ICRC), 38
International Council for Science (ICSU), 148, 149
International Strategy for Disaster Reduction (ISDR), 153
Intervention, 6, 13, 17, 20–22, 26, 27, 29, 41, 97–99, 101, 113, 162, 166, 170, 176, 177, 179, 180, 184, 193, 196, 197, 200
Interview, 7, 34, 112, 159, 166, 170, 171, 200
Iserson, K.V., 50
Israel Defense Forces Medical Corps, Haiti, 162

J
Jabbour, S., 184
Jaeschke, R., 98
Jafarey, A., 65
Japan 2011 earthquake and tsunami, 3, 18, 65, 96
Jewish Chronic Disease Hospital, 135
Jonas, H., 126
Jones, J., 131, 132
Joubert, G., 200
Just war theory, 28
Just war tradition, 27
Justice, 13, 25, 27, 28

K
Kahn, J., 113
Kaloupek, D.G., 200
Kanihan, S.F., 82
Kapp, C., 192, 199
Kar, N., 101
Kar-Purkayasha, I., 95, 100
Karadag, C.O., 5
Karma, 66
Kass, N.E., 50, 181
Katz, E., 82
Katz, J., 120, 133, 135
Kayabu, B., 97, 100
Keeton, C., 191
Kelly, E., 29
Khanna, R., 164
Kidnap, 24, 45
Kilpatrick, D.G., 200
King, N., 17, 199
King, N.B., 29
Klein, S., 6
Korf, B., 18
Kovats,S.R., 151
Kraul, M., 79
Kreiss, Y., 162
Kruger, F., 68
Kuhn, T.S., 97

L
Lakoff, A., 16, 17
Langer, E., 135
Largent, E.A., 110
Lay, T., 68
Lazarsfeld, P.F., 82
Leaning, J., 110, 120, 176
Lee, L.M., 5
Levine, C., 103, 164, 200
Lin, Y.A., 15

Lindell, M., 82
Loff, B., 100
Logistics, 17, 111
London, A.J., 138
Loyalty, 50, 53, 59
Luna, F., 166
Lurie, P., 136

M

Médecins Sans Frontières (MSF), 7, 10, 23, 113, 148, 168, 180
Macintyre, B., 19
Macklin, R., 170
Macro-ethics, 14
Magnuson, H.J., 134, 135
Magone, C., 5
Mahmud, S.M., 67, 103
Mahoney, J.F., 133, 134
Maiese, M., 145
Makgoba, W., 197
Malaria, 72, 133, 137
Malnutrition, 29, 119, 183, 197
Man-made disaster, 7, 10, 17, 18, 154, 192
  victims of, 24
Mandate, 28, 37, 43, 118
Martin, R., 74
Maschke, K.J., 117, 118
Mass-casualty disasters, 8
Masterson, L., 85
Mastrogianni, A., 66
Mayerfeld, J., 52
Mazzotta, M., 193
McClean, D., 3
McClement, S.E., 165
McKie, J., 146
McNeil, D.G., 130
Mead, R., 87
Measles, 72
Medicalization, 71
Men Who Stare at Goats, 129
Menikoff, J., 138
Meningitis study, 136
Meningitis treatment, 183
Merin, O., 33, 39, 50, 52, 59
Micro-ethics, 15, 17
Microbicide research, 198
Middleton, N., 18, 19, 21
Mifamurtide, 147
Miller, F., 113
Miller, P.B., 196
Minimal risk, 120, 135, 166, 171, 180, 182
Mississauga train derailment, 82
Molyneux, C.S, 200
Monitoring, 53, 109, 121, 125, 182
Moodley, K., 193–195, 197, 198, 200
Moral distress, 6, 8, 49
Moral failure, 43
Moral geography, 13, 18, 21, 22
Moral psychology, 55
Morphine, 54
Mouton, M., 192
Multi-drug resistant tuberculosis (MDR TB), 193
Murray, V., 154
Muslim, 66
Myer, L., 194

N

N-of-1 experiment, 41
Nardin, T., 23
Narrative, 55, 97
National Commission for the Protection of Human Subjects in Biomedical and Behavioral Research, 122
National Health Service (NHS), 144
National Institutes of Health (NIH), 132, 195
Natural
  victims of, 24
Natural disasters, 4, 10, 16–18, 26, 29, 37, 40, 50, 96, 150, 154, 167, 191
  groups of, 95
Natural hazard, 19
  impact of, 20
Needs assessment, 41, 73, 97, 102
Neutrality, 21, 38
  concept of, 21
  principle of, 23
Newberry, B., 19
Newman, E., 200
Ng, B.Y., 68
Niiler, E., 137
Non-intervention
  principle of, 22
Non-maleficence, 145
Nongovernmental organisation (NGO), 24, 27, 28, 67–69, 71, 73, 74, 110
Nuremberg code, 114, 115, 117, 122, 130, 132, 136

O

O'Mathúna, D.P., 41, 163, 165, 176
Oakes, J.M., 177
Obasogie, O.K., 123
Obligation, 5, 21, 26, 37, 38, 43, 66, 90, 110, 124, 125, 136, 169, 179, 186, 201
Ohrnberger, M., 68
Operational research, 6, 96, 113, 154, 182

Oppression, 38, 42
Orbinski, J., 39

P
Pakistan 2005 earthquake, 26
Palliation, 36
Palmer, I., 74
Pandey, B.N., 160
Pandolfi, M.M., 22, 24, 25
Parachute research, 194
Parfit, D., 58
Pasquali, S.K., 137
Pecoul, B., 180
Pellegrino, E.D., 14
Perrot, S., 23
Perry, R., 82
Pesik, N., 50
Peters, J.J., 136
Petrini, C., 15
Petryna, A., 137
Pfizer, 136
Pharmaceutical, 72, 124, 137, 146
Phase I trials, 121, 198
Philanthropic misconception, 67, 103, 119
Philanthropy, 22, 28
Philpott, S., 199
Photography, 52
Pitt, M., 151
Pittaway, E., 6
Placarding, 87–89
Placebo, 136, 195, 196, 198
Planning capacity, 17
Platt, C., 87
Pohlandt-McCormick, H., 192
Police, 53, 77, 82, 84, 90, 192
Political culture, 50
Political unrest, 192, 201
Post-traumatic stress disorder (PTSD), 101, 167
Poverty, 8, 19, 28, 29, 34, 96, 150, 167
Powerlessness, 43
Preparedness, 3, 16, 30, 41, 101, 124, 149, 153, 154, 162
  notion of, 17
  scope of, 17
Priority setting, 143, 144, 154
Prisoner, 122, 123, 125, 129, 131, 133, 134, 137, 164
Privacy, 52, 67, 78, 88, 89, 166
Professional capacity, 55
Psychological debriefing, 101
Public health, 5, 10, 16, 27, 29, 34, 36, 51, 53, 88, 113, 125, 131, 144, 150, 151, 162, 168, 169, 171, 181, 185, 188, 191, 193, 201
Public sympathy, 18

Q
Qualitative research, 6
Qualitative study, 34, 72
Quality of evidence, 98
Quality-adjusted life years (QALYs), 52
Quarantelli, E.L., 86, 101
Quarantine, 77, 79, 85, 88
Questionnaire, 112, 166, 169, 171

R
Rab, M.A., 181
Radiation accident, 160, 161
Rajpura, A., 100, 161
Randomised, 114, 162, 195, 198
Randomised controlled trial (RCT), 97
Rape, 113
Ravinetto, R., 187
Rawls, J., 50
Rawls, John, 50
Rechtman, R., 25
Reconstruction, 43, 153
Red Cross *See* International Committee of the Red Cross (ICRC), 23
Redmond, A.D., 100
Reductionism, 97
Redwood-Campbell, L.J., 37
Reed, H., 110
Refugee, 21, 22, 26, 113, 161, 164
Relevance, 72, 138, 145, 184
Religion, 67, 72, 101, 146
Research
  ethical guidelines for, 102
Research development, 169, 186, 194
Research ethics committee, 102, 104, 112, 152, 159, 168, 170, 171, 194
Resilience, 30, 71, 153
Resnik, D.B., 121
Respect for persons, 114, 116, 123
Responsibility, 7, 14, 18, 19, 29, 45, 50, 61, 181, 187
Responsiveness, 18, 41, 55
Reverby, S.M., 130–132
Reverse triage, 53
Revisability, 144
Reynolds, A., 83
Reynolds, B., 78
Rhabdomyolysis, 54, 61
Rhodes, R., 144
Richardson, J., 146
Rid, A., 119

Riddez, L., 37
Rinehart, A., 26
Risk, 3, 5, 6, 9, 19, 20, 45, 54, 61, 80, 82, 86, 88, 89, 96, 100, 109–118, 120, 121, 123, 126
Risk of bias, 98, 100
Roberts, I., 112
Roddy, R.E., 198
Rollins, N.C., 195
Rose, S., 71
Rose, S.C., 101
Rosenberg, C., 130
Rosenstein, D.L., 192, 200
Rossouw, T., 193
Roth, L.H., 165
Rothman, D.J., 122
Rule of rescue, 146
Russia 2010 heatwave, 3

S

Sabin, J.E., 144, 145
Sacred, 24, 126
Sacrificing, 24, 53
Safari research, 194
Samarasingha, D., 68
SAPIT trial, 198, 199
SARS epidemic, 113
Satcher, D., 136
Scanlon, J., 86
Scheid, D.E., 22
Schneider, C.E., 121
Schopper, D., 7, 104, 181
Schuklenk, U., 199
Schwartz, L., 6, 34–36, 39
Security, 7, 16, 17, 20, 26, 29, 45, 125, 137, 161
Seegar, M.W., 78, 81–83
Sekerka, L.E., 46
September 11th attacks (9/11), 50, 82, 166
Shah, T., 39, 148
Shamoo, A.E., 121
Shapiro, F., 71
Sheather, J., 39, 148
Shelter, 18, 21, 30, 59, 67, 68, 73, 74, 84, 161
Shuster, E., 115, 117, 129
Simmons, K., 84
Sims, H.J., 77
Siribaddana, S., 6, 67, 69, 73, 74
Siriwardana, C., 74
Siriwardhana, C., 194
Slim, H., 28, 29
Smith, M.J., 22
Smith, S., 131
Smith, W., 191, 192, 199
Social cohesion, 68
Social media, 77, 79, 84
Social science research, 165–167, 182, 193
Solbakk, J.H., 116, 117, 139
Son, W., 14
Sontag, D., 33
Sorokin, P.A., 52
South African disaster, 192
Sovereignty, 22, 26
Soweto riots, 1976, 192, 199
Sphere project, 2011, 38
Spokesperson, 82–84, 90
Sri Lanka, 8, 26, 65, 67–69, 72
Standards of care, 7, 51, 102, 104
Stein, R., 131
Stephens, M., 83
Stigmatised, 185
Stout, G.W., 132
Strength of recommendation, 98
Stress, 8, 35, 71, 165, 166, 200
Suffering, 7, 13, 18, 21, 24–26, 29, 49, 52, 54, 100, 149
Sumathipala, A., 6, 7, 47, 65, 67, 69, 71–74, 96, 102, 104, 179, 184
Surveillance, 109, 112, 113, 185
Survey, 6, 86, 112, 113, 125, 166, 170, 176, 182, 199
Symbolic consideration, 55
Sztajnkrycer, M.D., 15

T

Tabuchi, H., 111
Taking sides, 23
Tamiflu vaccine, 89
Tansey, C.M., 104, 179, 180, 183
Technological disaster, 17, 95
Ten Have, H., 14
Tessman, L., 42
Therapeutic illusion *See* philanthropic misconception, 119
Therapeutic misconception, 74, 103, 159, 183, 200
Thomson, J.J., 66
Three Mile Island, 83
Tornado, 84, 86
Torture, 129
Traditional healer, 67, 72
Transparency, 89–91, 138, 145, 146, 151
Tri-Council Policy Statement
  Ethical Conduct for Research Involving Humans, 178
Triage, 5, 8, 13, 15, 27, 36, 49, 52–59, 61, 162
  macro-triage, 13

micro-triage, 57
Trouiller, P., 180
Trovan meningitis study, 136, 137
Truman, Harry S., 21
Tschanz, D.W., 89
Twitter, 84

U
U.S. Code of Federal Regulations (CFR), 114
Ultra-orphan drugs, 146
Undue influence, 145, 163, 170, 184, 188
United Nations International Strategy for Disaster Reduction (UNISDR), 3
Unity, 21
Universal Declaration on Bioethics and Human Rights, 115, 116, 139
Universal Declaration on the Human Genome and Human Rights, 115
Universality, 21
Updegraff, J.A., 61
Upshur, R.E.G., 185
Utilitarian, 50, 52–55, 58, 61, 122, 123, 130
Utilitarian medicine, 53
Utilitarian scheme, 53
Utilitarian schemes, 59, 61
Utilitarianism, 54

V
Van Damme, L., 198
Varmus, H., 136, 196, 197
Victimhood, 25, 30
Vitamin A, 72
Volcanic ash, 151, 152
Volcanic eruption, 50
Voluntary, 21, 102, 115, 120, 168
Volunteers, 59, 80, 86, 87, 89, 134, 135, 148
Vromans, L., 192
Vulnerable, 9, 163, 164, 166, 167, 171, 172, 184, 198, 200
extrinsic vulnerability, 165, 166
intrinsic vulnerability, 165

W
Wallis, L., 191, 192, 199
Walzer, M., 22
Wang, T.L., 95, 101
War, 4, 17, 18, 21, 22, 26, 50, 71, 72, 86, 89, 109, 129, 130, 133, 138, 160, 184
Ward, R., 135
Watters, E., 68, 71–73
Weather-related disaster, 96
Weber, H., 151
Weiner, T., 130
Weiss, T.G., 21, 23, 28
Welfare, 10, 115, 121, 122, 129, 135, 136, 138, 159, 164, 167, 172
Well circumscribed disaster, 50, 51
Wendler, D., 114, 119
Wheeler, N.J., 22, 29
White, D.B., 53
White, M.M., 86
Whitney, S.N., 121
Williams, B., 62
Willitts-King, B., 98, 101
Willowbrook experiments, 135
Wilson, M., 112
Wilson, Woodrow, 21, 89
Witness bearing, 25
Wolinsky, H., 26, 27
Wood, E.B., 160, 171, 172, 176
Working Group on Disaster Research and Ethics (WGDRE), 102, 179
World bank, 99
World Health Organization (WHO), 17, 161

X
Xenophobic violence, 192, 199, 201

Y
Yamada, S., 69, 71
Yamout, R., 184

Z
Zack, N., 4
Zidovudine, 195–197
Zielinski, H., 39
Zwi, A.B., 176

Lightning Source UK Ltd.
Milton Keynes UK
UKHW022314190123
415646UK00005B/182

9 789400 738638